Practising social work

Social work in Britain today is currently being redefined in the face of new legislation on care in the community, the Criminal Justice Act and the Children Act. The wide range of methods of intervention now used by social workers means that the public at large expects clearer and more detailed explanation of social work approaches than ever before. Social workers will increasingly be called upon to explain to the public and users *what* they are doing and *how* they go about it.

Practising Social Work is a valuable contribution to the current debate on social work technique and method since it provides a systematic exploration of a range of social work approaches, with each chapter focusing on a single theme and explaining the practice implications of particular methods. Taking in a range of client groups, from young offenders to elderly people, the book includes chapters on anti-racist work, a feminist approach, and working with service users. Other chapters look at crisis intervention, alternatives to custody, family therapy, community work, systems theory, task-centred work, behaviourism, groupwork, casework, welfare rights, and contract work.

Practical in its approach, *Practising Social Work* will appeal to practitioners and students alike. It is designed to help social workers acquire greater professional knowledge, and to enable them to fulfil their prescribed roles, sensitive to their limitations but appropriately active in the service of the client. It will be essential reading for students and lecturers in social work and social policy, as well as for all professionals in the social work field.

Christopher Hanvey is director of the Thomas Coram Foundation, London and **Terry Philpot** is the editor of *Community Care* magazine.

Practising social work

Edited by Christopher Hanvey
and
Terry Philpot

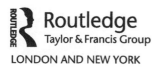

Routledge
Taylor & Francis Group

LONDON AND NEW YORK

by Routledge
on Park, Abingdon, Oxon, OX14 4RN
ue, New York, NY 10017

nt of the Taylor & Francis Group, an informa business

t and Christopher Hanvey, the collection as a
apters the contributors.

te names may be trademarks or registered trademarks,
for identification and explanation without intent to

loguing in Publication Data
or this book is available from the British Library.

Cataloging in Publication Data
vork/edited by Terry Philpot and Christopher

phical references and index.
- Great Britain. I. Philpot, Terry.
opher P.
4
0   93–28946
                                      CIP

/ Michael Mepham, Frome, Somerset.

-09236-4 (hbk)
-09237-1 (pbk)

To Rosemary and Mary

Contents

Contributors

Shama Ahmed was formerly a senior lecturer at the Polytechnic of North London, and is now a social work education adviser with CCETSW. She has worked as a probation officer, social worker and as a trainer and race policy adviser in the West Midlands. She has published widely.

Lorraine Ayensu is a health centre-based social worker for Avon Social Services Department in the central area of Bristol. Her professional interests include the promotion of anti-racist and anti-discriminatory social work policy and practice, and the empowerment of service users.

Peter Beresford is a member of Survivors Speak Out, and senior lecturer in social policy at the West London Institute of Higher Education. Since 1987 he has worked with the Open Services Project, funded by the Joseph Rowntree Foundation, to help people gain more say in their lives and in the services they use.

Allan Brown is a senior lecturer in social work at Bristol University. He is the author of *Groupwork* (now in its third edition), and co-editor of the journal *Groupwork*, which he co-founded in 1988. His interests include anti-discrimination in relation to groupwork, and groupwork in the criminal justice system.

Paul Burgess is principal welfare rights officer for Lancashire County Council. Before training in the social sciences he worked in engineering from leaving school, and became active nationally in trade union affairs. As well as broadcasting on TV and radio, he has tutored welfare rights courses for many years, and written widely on the subject, including a column for the magazine *Community Care* since 1979.

Suzy Croft is a qualified and practising social worker. She has a long-standing involvement in issues of participation and empowerment as a researcher, service user and through her involvement in community action. With Peter Beresford, she has worked with the Open Services Project since 1987.

Mark Doel is a lecturer in social work at Sheffield University and a freelance trainer. During 1990–91 he directed a research project as part of the Families as Allies programme at Portland State University, Oregon. His book, *Task-Centred Social Work*, co-authored with Peter Marsh, is the most recent summary of task-centred practice in Britain.

Celia Doyle is a senior lecturer in social work and a freelance practitioner and consultant. For many years she has specialized in work with abused children and their families. She has published on a variety of issues relating to child protection and is involved in research on the emotional abuse of children.

Christopher Hanvey is director of the Thomas Coram Foundation. He has a career in social welfare, both in the statutory and voluntary sectors. He is author of a book on learning disabilities, has written for the Open University, and contributes regularly to a range of journals.

Annie Hudson is a team manager with Avon Social Services Department working in the central area of Bristol. She was formerly a lecturer in social work at Manchester University. Her research and professional interests have included social work with young women, child abuse, and social work management.

Marjorie Mayo is a tutor at Ruskin College, Oxford. Apart from teaching and research, she has previously worked on a women's employment and training project, and with community and trade union organizations. She has worked in local government, and was a research officer on the government's Community Development Project and the European Community's second anti-poverty programme. She has published widely.

Catherine Oadley qualified as a social worker in 1988 and now works with Avon Social Services Department in the central area of Bristol. Her professional interests include child protection work, and therapeutic and direct work with children and adult women.

Kieran O'Hagan is a lecturer in social work at The Queen's University, Belfast. He was a front line social work practitioner for fifteen years. He has worked in Mother Teresa's establishments in Calcutta and Los Angeles, and lectured on crisis intervention and child abuse in Australia. He has written numerous articles and books on crisis intervention and child abuse, and more recently, has concentrated on training and writing about the crises of child sexual abuse.

Matilde Patocchi qualified as a social worker in 1990, and now works with Avon Social Services Department in the central area of Bristol. Her professional interests have included child protection and family placement work.

Chris Payne is Consultant in Social Care at the National Institute for Social Work, and co-Director of the Centre for Practice and Staff Development based at the University of Warwick Science Park. Much of his earlier work was spent on examining the application of unitary perspective to UK social services and social work education. He has a particular interest in the application of general systems theory to residential care, reflected in his numerous publications.

Terry Philpot is Editor of *Community Care*. He has published work on several aspects of social work, and is currently writing a book about the National Children's Home. He is an honorary member of the council of the NSPCC, and formerly a member of the advisory council of the Centre for Policy on Ageing.

John Pierson worked as a social worker in both field and residential settings. He subsequently became Senior Training Officer and Training Manager with Cheshire Social Services and now teaches part-time at Staffordshire University. He is also a training consultant and is currently working on a dictionary of social care and social work.

Michael Preston-Shoot is Senior Lecturer in social work at the University of Manchester, School of Social Work. He is also a psychotherapist and family therapist.

Philippa Seligman is a family therapist in private practice as a clinician and trainer in Cardiff, where she lives, and in London. She was a member of the internationally recognized team at the Family Institute in Cardiff and has numerous publications to her credit. In 1991 she was elected chairperson of the Association for Family Therapy in the UK for a three-year term of office.

Norman Tutt originally trained as a clinical psychologist and has direct experience of working in the N. H. S. During the 1970s he was responsible for the planning of children's services for the 33 London Boroughs. From 1975 – 79 he was adviser to the Secretary of State for Health and Social Security. In 1979 he became Professor of Applied Social Studies at the University of Lancaster and from 1988 to 1992 was Director of Social Services, Leeds City Council. In 1992 he left Leeds to return to Social Information Systems Ltd, a consultancy he had founded ten years previously. He is the author of a number of books and articles on social policy.

Acknowledgements

An edited collection must, by definition, be more of a collective effort than a book by one author. As editors we would like to thank the contributors for their hard work, achieved by all of them while undertaking demanding professional responsibilities; for meeting their various deadlines, and for responding, without quarrel, to our suggestions for changes, both large and small.

We should like to thank especially Martin Davies, director of the social work programme, University of East Anglia, whose original suggestions, longer ago than we care to remember, helped shape the book and brought to our attention some of the contributors. We should also like to thank Linda Ward of the Norah Fry Research Centre, University of Bristol, and John Pierson for their helpful comments on our introduction. Last, and by no means because tradition dictates, any errors and omissions must reside with us.

Christopher Hanvey and
Terry Philpot

Introduction

Terry Philpot and Christopher Hanvey

Social work is what social workers do. The old humorous definition contains more than an element of truth. It might be reworked to explain that social work is often what others – nurses, doctors, the police, and so on – don't do. Just as social work often picks up the casualties where society – in its housing, employment, anti-poverty policies – has failed, so often it assumes the tasks arising where other agencies – medical and nursing services, the police – do not tread. But social work may be defined in other ways. Social work is casework, declared Robert Pinker in his dissenting note to the Barclay report (Pinker 1982). Or social work may be defined by its legislative responsibilities. This latter, though, is less a definition of what social workers do, other than in a very functional sense, than drawing the boundaries at their legal obligations. The burden of legislation does, indeed, lie heavily on social work, and increasingly so, yet there are numerous tasks which social workers undertake for which there is no specific legislative remit.

This book is not an explicit attempt to define social work, but rather to explain the theory and practice of a number of social work methods. Social work has always adopted a range of methods of work or approaches. Some of these have been generated by the organizational structures within which social work is situated, some by sociological theory which has emerged alongside day-to-day practice. The approach, for example, described in George Konrad's novel *The Caseworker* (Konrad 1987), whereby 'one of us will talk, the other will listen', has a growing literature and, despite its obvious affiliation with counselling (Halmos 1965), can encompass a multitude of methods of working in which the exploration of problems at a one-to-one level hopefully engenders new insight and a way through what may seem like intractable problems. Celia Doyle, one of the contributors to this book, describes the honourable history of casework and stresses the consistent value placed on the individual as being basic to any kind of practice.

Yet, the language with which social work seeks even to describe the jobs which its members undertake is often obfuscatory. In 1978 Barbara Wootton drew attention to this fact by considering recruitment advertisements for social workers. She wrote:

> ... one such [advertisement] asks for qualified applicants who are used to 'statutory duties' and have the ability to 'act independently and take appropriate decisions' (about what?). Another mentions that the successful applicant will be expected to 'work with families and children' (on what?); and yet another asks for an 'intake social worker' to 'join a team' which is 'developing systems and methods useful to clients and staff'.
>
> (Wootton 1978).

She went on: 'The layman may well be puzzled to visualise how the holders of these posts will spend their working hours.' That was then. What would she say now, given the frequent replacement of the title 'social worker' by 'project leader', 'key worker', 'care manager' and a dozen other not very self-explanatory variants?

In fairness, many professional self-descriptions may be criticized in this way, containing a salad of esoteric language and jargon. Social work, however, labours under a particular challenge since, as a discipline, it has absorbed the professional language of psychology, psychiatry, sociology, politics and medicine. This creates a particular responsibility to define terms carefully, a discipline imposed on all the authors of the present volume.

Martin Davies (1985) has also drawn attention to another problem for social work. He was at first (1981) taken with Olive Stevenson's belief that social workers are 'brokers in shades of grey', when she wrote:

> Those who commit themselves to social work contribute, in my view, to the sensitisation of our society. In doing so, they will not be popular.... They must seek to hold, and to mediate in, the multiplicity of conflict in interpersonal relationships. They deal in shades of grey where the public looks for black and white. And they are bitterly resented for it. They are brokers in lesser evils, frequently faced with the need for choice followed by action whose outcome is unpredictable. In the precise sense of the word, society is deeply ambivalent about social work, asking it more and more to combat the alienation of a technological age, yet resenting its growing power and quick to point harshly to its failures, especially those in relation to functions of social control.
>
> (Stevenson 1974)

For Davies that statement nearly ten years ago

> ... so nearly hits the nail on the head in its attempt to identify the reason for the public's disaffection with social work; it so nearly scores a

bull's-eye in its assessment of the role of social work in society, and the function which social work fulfils as society's insurance against alienation; and it does succeed in its account of the way in which the social work process is a dynamic one, always moving, never finished, operating constantly against a back cloth of uncertainty and external influence.

(Davies 1981)

Yet when Davies came to revise his book four years later he regarded Stevenson's 'brokers in shades of grey' as 'a seductive phrase' and dispensed entirely with his chapter on the subject. Recanting his past attraction, he wrote:

Social workers have no monopoly of such a role, and too often the idea can be misconstrued and used self-indulgently to justify indecision, buck-passing and theoretical squeamishness. The truth is that social workers are employed to do a wide-ranging but quite specific job, which necessarily involves them in risk-taking, decision making and the exercise of judgement. They cannot expect always to be right or regularly to receive public plaudits. But they should nonetheless determine to be knowledgeable in relevant spheres, adept at fulfilling their ascribed roles, sensitive to personal and occupation limitations, and appropriately active in service of the client.

(Davies 1985)

Davies is, we believe, right to suggest that Stevenson's view has sometimes acted as a camouflage for the shortcomings he lists. However, we do not believe that there is a conflict between the situation she so eloquently describes and the need to see social workers as having a 'wide-ranging but quite specific job'. Being 'brokers in shades of grey' is, arguably, a consequence of having to deal with the rough and unpredictable material of humanity. Martin Davies himself has written of

... the frailties of human genetics and the ageing body... the aberrations of human behaviour... plans [that] go wrong and people die... all political and economic systems... produce victims and label deviants... human nature and human life are occasionally vicious, and... people – especially in families – sometimes fight and hurt each other.

(Davies 1981)

The problems social workers face are not so neatly dealt with as are problems faced by professionals who have to hand the arrest, the fire hose or the scalpel. The material clues, the heart beat, and the pulse, are, whatever the problems faced by others, more specific and scientific than what is often available to social workers.

This book is very much about assisting the acquisition of professional knowledge, and helping practitioners to fulfil their prescribed roles, to help them to be 'sensitive to personal and professional limitations, and [to be] appropriately active in the services of the client', as Davies counsels. But in deciding which methods to include we came upon problems of definition. Some readers may dispute whether the areas of practice we have included here are, indeed, social work at all: welfare rights and community work among them. Yet these two fields are so inextricably involved with contemporary social work that no damage is done to them, nor to social work, we believe, by making our definition broad enough to include them.

Marjorie Mayo shows that community work is subject to varied definitions. It is also practised within other local authority departments, like housing, as well as outside local government altogether. With regard to welfare rights, Paul Burgess believes that it is not strictly social work and that there are many reasons why social workers cannot undertake it. His view is that in twenty years it has grown to a specialism of its own, sometimes organizationally placed within social services and social work departments, and sometimes not, assisting social workers in their rightful concern with clients' welfare rights. Norman Tutt asks if alternatives to custody as an approach is social work, while John Pierson says of behaviourism that what suits the clinician does not necessarily suit the social worker.

We have not seen social work as a vertical activity. Chris Payne's chapter on a systems approach, for example, argues for less reliance on casework and a one-to-one approach, opting instead for working through teams, groups, and, if necessary, communities. Similarly, other approaches have cut across traditional divisions and operate in a variety of ways, as Annie Hudson, Lorraine Ayensu, Catherine Oadley and Matilde Patocchi, and Shama Ahmed show with regard to feminism and anti-racism, respectively. (However, Hudson, Ayensu, Oadley and Patocchi, in particular, are careful to emphasize the dangers of a narrow, exclusive definition of a feminist approach, which may too rigidly define the root of the problems faced by a client.) Likewise, crisis intervention may be just as useful with groups as with individuals. It recognizes that the twin natures of crisis are danger and opportunity, which provide the most profitable time to intervene in situations. In his exploration of crisis intervention, Kieran O'Hagan is careful to emphasize that no method of social work can be divorced from its ethical context, and while crisis may provide the most fruitful time for intervention, consideration needs to be given to whether this is ethically justified. For Philippa Seligman family therapy embraces both the personal and the collective. Allan Brown has sought to demystify the idea of groupwork by a comprehensive definition, embracing community groups, as well as personal therapy groups of half a dozen or so members. Thus, he not only marries the various strands of groupwork but the diverse traditions of social work itself.

Just as social work draws on the language of other professions, so too do its methods of intervention sometimes owe a debt to other professions. A contract approach to social work, for example, described by Michael Preston-Shoot, attempts to break down barriers between the power of the 'expert' and the feelings of powerlessness experienced by those seeking help. The contract, it is argued, allows for a more equal relationship between helper and helped. Here, there are similarities and overlap with task-centred work, which Mark Doel characterizes as being based on partnership and empowerment for the mutual definition of problems.

Our intention, then, has been to provide an inclusive systematic exploration of the range of social work approaches. Each chapter provides a basic description and discussion of the approach, exploring the implications, with examples from practice, as well as offering a critique. Social work is perhaps less prone these days to make too many immodest claims about its ability to cure all the world's ills, but we have thought it important that a critical edge be given to each chapter.

This book is aimed at practitioners as much as students. It is not envisaged that any worker would adopt one approach exclusively. We hope it develops a catholic approach which, in its totality, recognizes the contribution that a wide range of approaches have made to practice. This latter point should be emphasized. Social work's roots are, as we have said, diverse. But there can be a danger, as well as a strength in eclecticism where a method is adopted for work with an individual or family because the worker has a penchant for it rather than because it has been shown to provide better results. Evidence for this has come in Kathryn Ellis's study of assessment (Ellis 1993). Observing assessors and disabled users during assessments, she found that some social workers, attached to psychological explanations and counselling techniques, would diagnose users' needs not on the basis of how the user perceived them – for example, for equipment or practical assistance – but on the basis of their own professional predilections. For example, some social workers tended to see physical impairment in terms of loss and bereavement. People who became disabled were thought to be going through a grieving process for which the practitioner required special skills. In one case sight loss had radically altered the life of an older woman. Having had an active social life and having never felt lonely, she now lacked the self-confidence to go out alone. Afraid that her sight would further deteriorate and depressed at her situation, she lost weight which meant that her clothes no longer fitted. Once proud of her smart and youthful appearance, she would no longer visit friends, thus compounding her isolation. The social worker believed that her case constituted a 'hierarchy of losses' in which, as Ellis explains, 'the traumatic loss of a parent was the most fundamental and unresolved issue. The practitioner theorised that, although the loss of sight had become the focus for other losses, it was actually the least significant'. The rehabilitation officer, unencumbered by all this theory, believed that mobility training – for which the woman lacked confidence – would assist her, diagnosing that the lack of social contact was the main issue. The social worker, however, thought that she was 'emotionally housebound', believing her to be more capable than she claimed, and thus doubting the usefulness of mobility training. The woman (we might think surprisingly) was appreciative of all these efforts, but what she really wanted was someone to take her out occasionally, especially for shopping. She, too, had not read the right books on social work theory! Eclecticism in that context debilitates any usefulness it might have, is unhealthy and becomes a dog's dinner – and a pretty inedible one at that.

It is arguable that there is a certain luxury in offering such descriptions as does this book in the light of the current changes facing social work, particularly the advent of community care. Allan Brown is not the only contributor to find the thrust of social services and social work departments and the climate within which they operate to be unsympathetic to his subject, groupwork. To take another area, community work ought to be coming into its own with its long-standing and inherent emphasis on user involvement. But cuts in voluntary sector funding and the feared trend that some voluntary agencies may become little more than arms of statutory services may work against this.

Suzy Croft and Peter Beresford argue that the new role of care manager and the creation of a care market run the risk of combining the shortcomings of both the state and market systems, with services provided for cash, not need, and needs being defined by professionals, rather than by service users themselves. Under the new arrangements, the central figure will be the care manager. The consumer in this arrangement is not the purchaser: the purchaser is the social services or health authority. The new mixed economy of care, with its purchaser/provider split, contracting, packages of care and care management has been ushered in ostensibly because it was believed that social services and social work departments were monolithic providers, whose services did not meet individual needs. The reforms have allegedly been posited on the needs of the user. 'The rationale for these reforms is the empowerment of users and carers', declared the government (Social Services Inspectorate 1991), drawing on the example of the commercial market place as a means of meeting individual need and ensuring choice. But there is no certainty that the objectives of greater choice for users will be met (Common and Flynn 1992); in care managers, users may well meet (to pursue the market analogy) not an assistant who helps them to purchase the goods they want, but an officious shopkeeper who tells them what he or she has on their shelf irrespective of their needs, a replica of the worst present practice (see Ellis 1993).

The new market of care may not just change the role of the social worker (or add a new approach!) but may even exclude social workers from what will be a central role within social services and social work departments. The responsibilities of assessment, service co-ordination, acting as a go-between for suppliers and the purchasing authority, holding budgets and creating care packages are not those traditionally associated with social work, and are certainly a far cry from Konrad's 'one of us will talk, the other will listen'. Sir Roy Griffiths in his germinative report on the future of community care (Griffiths 1988) made no reference to social workers, and already care managers are being recruited from outside the ranks of social work, for example from home help organizers, whose own skills are more in tune with those required by the care manager.

But if social workers are to retain a central role in the new arrangements, they must avoid the shortcoming which Wootton described. In the coming contract culture social workers will be called upon more than ever to explain to the public and users what it is they are doing and how they go about it. A discussion of technique and method is therefore timely.

And so this book appears when social work is again redefining itself (or being redefined!) in the wake of the Children Act, the Criminal Justice Act, and the NHS and Community Care Act. The need for greater clarity about ways of working and what social workers do has never been stronger. We have tried to offer that clarity.

REFERENCES

Common, R. and Flynn, N. (1992) *Contracting for Care*, York: Joseph Rowntree Foundation/*Community Care*.
Davies, M. (1981) *The Essential Social Worker*, London: Heinemann Educational Books/*Community Care*. Second edn (1985), Aldershot: Gower/*Community Care*.
Ellis, K. (1993) *Squaring the Circle: User and Carer Participation in Need Assessment*, York: Joseph Rowntree Foundation/*Community Care*.
Griffiths, Sir Roy (1988) *Community Care: Agenda for Action*, London: HMSO.
Halmos, P. (1965) *The Faith of the Counsellors*, London: Constable.
Konrad, G. (1987) *The Caseworker*, Harmondsworth: Penguin.
Pinker, R. (1982) 'An alternative view', in Barclay Committee, *Social Workers: Their Roles and Tasks*, London: National Institute for Social Work/Bedford Square Press.
Social Services Inspectorate (1991) *Care Management and Assessment: Managers' Guide*, London: HMSO.
Stevenson, O. (1974) Editorial, *British Journal of Social Work* 4(1), Spring.
Wootton, B. (1978) 'The social work task today', *Community Care*, 4 October.

1 The systems approach

Chris Payne

Interest in the application of systems theory to social work gathered momentum in the late 1950s and 1960s (e. g. Buckley 1967, Hearn 1968) and reached its height with the publication of major American texts by Howard Goldstein and Pincus and Minahan in 1973. These and other texts that proclaimed a 'unitary' perspective were used widely on social work training courses in the UK during the 1970s and beyond together with the important 'bridging' text of Specht and Vickery, *Integrating Social Work Methods* (1977).

When first introduced, the systems approach was regarded not just as a conceptual framework, but also as a symbol of unification that would promote the incipient power and influence of the social work profession. Here it needs to be noted that the approach was introduced at an early stage of development of the new monolithic social services departments and of 'integrated' social work training (i. e. CQSW) courses. These developments required some common, unifying principles to underpin the methods of service delivery of the new 'generic' social workers. Such principles were articulated in a variety of publications on unitary approaches. Not all unitary perspectives used systems theory for underpinning, however, and certainly there has never been any wholesale and uncritical adoption by social work training of either a systems or a unitary approach.

The other pressure for integration, which the systems approach was expected to assist, was of the methods and techniques at the disposal of social workers, notably casework, groupwork and community work, and arguably residential work (Payne 1977). The approach provided a means by which a wide range of interventive methods, including some based on opposing treatment ideologies and theories such as behavioural and psychodynamic methods, could be differentially and acceptably employed within a comprehensive unitary model of social work.

In brief, systems theory historically has made three major contributions to social work developments.

1 To provide the basis for a unified profession of social work; this has certainly not been achieved.

2 To provide an overarching and permeating theory for social work practice. This, as we will see, has been problematical to say the least.

3 To assist with the integration of the different traditions and methods that have characterized social work, i. e. casework, groupwork, residential work and community work; and of the different academic disciplines that inform social work, i. e. sociology, psychology, social policy, etc. How effective this has been is also difficult to evaluate.

The history is important because the systems approach has now lost much of its potency to stimulate debate and controversy and little of substance has been written on it over the past few years. It may still be referred to and used in social work training and practice; for example, implicitly in relation to the community social work approach (Smale *et al.* 1988) and explicitly in some forms of family therapy (e. g. Minuchin 1974). There is an excellent systems analysis of residential practice by Atherton (1989). Systems concepts are also implicit in 'ecological' and 'social networking' models (e. g. Davies 1977, Whittaker and Garbarino 1983). However, it would seem that social work has to a large extent lost its taste for 'grand theory', which the approach represented, and for the political interventions and confrontational style which were seen to follow from a systems analysis of social needs and problems.

During the 1970s the systems approach provoked quite passionate debates between its proponents and antagonists. For example, one critical article by Bill Jordan, which appeared in *New Society* in 1977, provoked such a furore that a special correspondence page had to be given over to the responses. The approach was criticized by Marxists because it appeared too conservative and offered little analysis of the structural causes of personal distress and difficulty. It was criticized by traditionalists because it allegedly took social work away from its roots of helping individuals and made social work an impersonal and bureaucratized set of activities. Alternatively it could be criticized because it potentially took social workers into the political arena and into confrontations with, for example, the employing agencies.

Some criticisms of the approach were based on a misunderstanding of the role of systems theory, which was less that of a comprehensive 'grand theory' of society on a par with, say, Marxism, than that of a 'meta theory' that could help social workers organize and integrate different perspectives and methods for achieving relatively small-scale personal and social changes.

There are several possible explanations as to why the systems approach is today deemed less fashionable and tendentious. First, in recent years, as a response to criticisms of so-called 'generic work', and coming mainly as a result of the series of child abuse scandals and inquiries, there has been a growing trend to return to specialization by client group. With the implementation of the 1989 Children Act and 1990 NHS Community Care Act with its 'purchasing/providing' divisions, specialization is likely to increase further. These trends towards greater specialization are correspondingly reflected in the changes to qualifying social work training and the new Diploma in Social Work regulations. They do not, it should be stated, invalidate the systems approach, but may make it more difficult to apply.

The application of a unitary model has also been affected by other factors: ideological pressure from the Right to reduce 'welfarism'; changes in legislation and procedures, particularly in relation to child protection, which have increased the social policing role of the social worker; and resource constraints and other financial pressures on the main employers of social workers, the local authorities, which have resulted in an erosion of the 'resource systems' available to social workers. The scenario of the 1990s is one of mainstream social work becoming, if anything, more conservative, procedural and managerial, in effect returning to its historical role of helping individuals as opposed to achieving radical social change through systemic action. In *The Essential Social Worker* Davies perhaps represents most clearly what social work has in fact become, when he argues that the main function of social work is not the achievement of large-scale social change, which is implicit in some unitary approaches. Its role is rather that of *maintenance*. 'Social workers are the maintenance mechanics oiling the interpersonal wheels of the community' (Davies 1981: 137).

Given the current state of social work, a renewal of interest in the systems approach could be no bad thing. I state this because the profession appears to have become sadly fragmented and to have lost its vision of the kind of society that would seem to follow from the articulation and application of its values. It is true that there is currently a great deal of 'issue-raising' about equal opportunities, anti-oppressive and anti-discriminatory practice, but few well thought out strategies to realize these goals. The systems approach does not have all the solutions here, but it does have the merit of offering a way of analysing and thinking through these issues and identifying appropriate strategies for action.

The systems approach also acts as a conceptual framework, which can reduce theoretical fragmentation. For example in a recent study of student placement records covering nine CQSW courses, it was stated there 'was no evidence at all of the consistent or systematic application of a particular framework, approach or theory. Where theorising did appear to be taking place it was on a piecemeal basis with no overall strategy or tactic discernible' (Thompson 1991).

THE SYSTEMS APPROACH

For a much fuller description and critique than can be offered here, the reader is referred to M. Payne (1991). Here we provide a simple guide for getting to grips with a fairly complicated set of ideas (which could also explain its unpopularity!).

The basis of the systems approach and its understanding lies in social systems theory. Thus to start with we need a definition of a social system. Buckley's is generally considered to be helpful:

> A complex of elements or components directly or indirectly related in a causal network, such that each component is related to at least some others in a more or less stable way within a particular period of time.
>
> (Buckley 1967: 41)

This definition can thus be used in relation to:

- human beings as biological and psychological systems;
- simple social relationships, e. g. couples whose actions and behaviour will invariably need to be explained in relation to one another: *A*'s behaviour towards *B* being determined by *B*'s behaviour towards *A* through their continuing interaction. Thus an explanation of the behaviour of one cannot be made without reference to the other, not as separate individuals, but taken together as an entity. A 'symbiotic relationship', for example, is one that can only be explained systemically;
- nuclear and extended families and kinship networks;
- neighbourhoods and social networks, organizations and associations of different sorts, e. g. community groups, political parties, Round Table, etc.
- work organizations, local authorities, voluntary agencies, etc.
- the civil service, the government, the world, the universe, etc.

The assumption made in describing any social organization as a 'system' is that behaviour, events and social processes cannot be fully understood in isolation, but only in relation to one another. Systemic influences may be direct and indirect; connections may not be obvious but could arguably be identified from research and analysis. For example the composition and culture of, say, a particular middle-class residential neighbourhood, is clearly not created from 'individual choice' alone. It will be influenced, for example, by the range and style of houses, and the planning processes that have been employed, which will determine their price and therefore who can afford to live there. Some income groups (and social classes) will therefore be excluded from taking up residence there. Many of the influences on people's lives are covert or indirect, such as the economic and political, but when analysed systemically can be identified and weighed up accordingly.

The emphasis in systems theory on interactions, transactions, context, interrelatedness, and the idea that the sum total is greater than the individual parts certainly shifts attention away from 'disease' and 'pathological' theories of behaviour towards multi-causal, interactional explanations (Triseliotis 1978). Social systems theory is itself a progression from *general systems theory* postulating that all phenomena or events – physical, chemical, biological or social – should be conceptualized as organized wholes or entities, where the components are functionally interrelated as subsystems. Each system is thus interconnected with others occurring in its total environment (von Bertalanffy *et al.* 1951).

General systems are of four main types:

1 *Natural* systems such as the universe or solar system; life systems in terms of their anatomy, physiology, biology and ecology.
2 *Physical design* systems, e. g. engineering, central heating, gas distribution, motor car engine systems.
3 *Abstract design* systems such as mathematical and computer language systems.
4 *Human activity* systems, i. e. social organizations like families and the Girl Guides.

One of the problems for social work is the limitations of theories about social systems, which are not as advanced as in other disciplines, engineering for example. Systems can be thought of as being 'hard' or 'soft'. Analysis of a fault occurring in a 'hard' system, for example a motor car engine, can be undertaken systematically on the assumption that sooner or later it will be located and diagnosed. This is because there is a body of knowledge to explain the working of the whole system and its parts. Social systems are problematical because there is rarely the same kind of 'hard' knowledge – such is the status of the social compared to the natural sciences – to account for their operations. Consequently there must inevitably be more recourse to conjecture and speculation about individual situations, and evidence collection and appraisal on which to base an assessment is made much more difficult. Triseliotis (1978), for example, has criticized the application of systems theory to social work for being too vague and generalized and of little practical value, because it is impossible to predict from it what is likely to have occurred or will happen in specific instances.

Where attempts are made to describe social systems as if they are capable of being 'hard', criticism is then levelled that the model of society is overly mechanistic and reductionist. One of the common criticisms of the systems approach from the Left has always been that it assumes a static, Parsonian model of social structure and process, in which society is regarded more as a closed than an open system. This is not a valid criticism of systems theory as such, but only of a particular interpretation of it, the structural–functionalist approach. It is based on a partial understanding of types of systems, which are more likely within the concept of general systems to be characterized by fluidity, flexibility and potential for change on many levels.

Indeed, one of the problems of the systems approach is that almost anything can be defined as a system to the point where it becomes meaningless to do so. For example, it is pointless to use the concepts of 'change agent', 'client', 'target' and 'action' *systems* as in the Pincus and Minahan model (the best known of the unitary approaches), unless systems features and processes are actually understood and used to make social work assessments and to identify the interventions that should logically follow. My reading of many students' essays and assignments over the years suggests that what has often been missing has been a good grasp of 'systems thinking' and its practical implications; all that is learned is a facile relabelling of more traditional approaches and a continuation of existing styles of working.

Thinking 'systemically' means that many influences that are not obviously included in an assessment of a 'problem' will be so. For example, if we were to examine the performance of a social work team, one approach would be to assess the performance of individual team members solely in relation to their job descriptions and other formal organizational expectations. A team viewed as a social system, as an entity whose components interrelate, will suggest a different assessment approach. Here we would need to explore how the variables associated with roles, power and influence, team values and culture, gender and race, amongst others, all interact and contribute to how the team is operating as a *whole* and *then* look at the effects on individual members. The interconnectedness of the different 'subsystems' will be demonstrated when, for example, the power of some individual team members will be identified as a source of stress for others. This in turn may create conflict and unhealthy tensions in working relationships and erode the team's accepted value base. Once the analysis has been completed in systems terms, the appropriate actions may follow. For example, the team might decide to review its values and goals, from which new or modified plans of action are identified that begin to address the imbalances that have been identified in working relationships (see also Douglas and Payne 1989).

However, thinking systemically may give the feeling of operating on shifting sands. This is partly because the definition of a 'social system', i. e. in terms of its purpose, structure, boundaries, processes and so on, will vary according to the *perspective* from which it is defined. A 'helping system', for example, may be defined differently for a field social worker than for a residential worker or foster parent, despite the fact that they all share a common concern – a child or children in care. One might assume that all have a common purpose – the welfare and interests of the child. However, the perspective of the field social worker may well conflict with those of the residential worker or foster parents, and where they do, difficulties in identifying and therefore achieving goals can easily be predicted. Work has to be done, therefore, between those involved to create *common* definitions of the goals and tasks so that a *common* perspective is being followed and all recognize that they are operating within *common* (system) boundaries.

KEY CONCEPTS OF SYSTEMS THEORY

There are a limited number of key concepts that have to be grasped, without which it is impossible to apply any model of practice founded on a systems theory, including, for example, certain family therapy approaches. I shall describe these as simply as I can.

Basic characteristics

All systems, by definition, have *boundaries* that differentiate them from their environment and other systems, though there may be considerable overlaying of one system on another. In social systems the boundaries are always permeable to some extent; in other words, they can be penetrated at different points. The more permeable the boundary the more open and flexible the system is said to be. Compare a prison, as an example of a relatively closed type of system, with a drop-in centre as an example of a more open system. How open and closed a system needs to be to operate effectively again will depend on the circumstances. Even the universe is no longer regarded as a completely closed and bounded system. Closed systems lose their means of drawing in energy across their boundaries and they die, for example as when a group of people marooned on a desert island lose their supply and means of producing food and water.

Operations

'Input', 'throughput' (conversion or transformation), 'output' and 'feedback' are the technical terms used.

    Input is what you must put into a system to make it work, for example, human, physical, material and financial resources must be contributed in the right ways and right amounts to achieve the results required. The 'human' inputs may be described in terms of numbers, time and effort, roles and skills, communications, etc., depending on the system in question. Clearly imbalances between the different kinds of resources needed will affect how well the system can perform and there will be all sorts of knock-on effects. Good parenting is not helped by having no money. Being short staffed puts pressures on people so that they may not be able to deliver the sort of service they want to give. Lack of secretarial or clerical help may mean more time having to be spent on paperwork and less on direct work with clients.

Throughput is how the resources are used in their entirety to achieve the desired results, for example, what happens after the petrol has been put in and the engine started up. The problem with social systems is that we do not really know sufficiently well how or why things happen as they do. Try to fathom out the real causes of a disruption in a residential setting, for example, and one often starts with a mish-mash of inconsistent and contradictory information. It is only by evaluating the information and relating it to a host of possible interconnected causes that something approaching a satisfactory explanation begins to emerge. No single explanation or cause is ever likely to be valid.

Outputs are the results that you have achieved, the success of which can then be evaluated against the original goals. Evaluation of effectiveness is of course problematical in social work, not least because it is virtually impossible to identify, control and evaluate every factor that contributes to a particular outcome. Evaluation, in systems terms, means identifying the main inputs (needed to achieve stated goals), assessing how these have been converted into practical action (processes), and similarly appraising what results have been achieved, taking all factors into account, not as isolated variables, but interrelatedly.

Feedback is the information and messages received back at different stages in the process. Because of the lack of predictability of social work it is important to obtain feedback continuously so that adjustments can be made that will help to keep one on track. The feedback received can then be used and reconverted as further inputs. This is the basis of good management information and monitoring processes.

Systems processes

The key words are 'steady state' or 'equilibrium', 'reverberation', 'equifinality', 'multifinality' and 'differentiation'.

Steady state is the tendency of systems to maintain themselves in some sort of balance while at the same time moving forwards towards their goals. Systems can be knocked off balance or continue to operate in less than optimum ways, as in a state of chronic depression. Imbalances may be caused by all sorts of things such as deficits of resources, disturbances and breakdowns of parts or all of the system. The effects are sometimes cumulative, for example: loss of job → lack of money → lowering of morale and self-esteem → increased debt → impaired personal relationships → 'uncharacteristic' behaviour → total crisis.

Reverberation means knock-on effects, which can be far reaching, though the causal path may be difficult to establish. For example, loss of job → lowered self-esteem, reinforced further by failure to meet expectations developed from childhood → depression. In this example the links with the person's past may take some time to establish.

Equifinality means that the same results may be reached in different ways and through different routes.

Multifinality means that different results may be obtained in ostensibly similar circumstances because differences in *process* may have occurred, i.e. parts of the system have interacted in different ways. This is quite common in social work, because of the difficulty in identifying and controlling within an intervention plan all of the variables involved.

Differentiation is the means by which systems maintain their 'identity' through the regulation and operation of their boundaries.

AN EXAMPLE OF THE APPLICATION OF A SYSTEMS APPROACH

Rather than dwell on the concepts we can illustrate how a systems approach can be used in practice. Here we use the approach as a set of tools for assessment and planning interventions. The example is not intended to demonstrate any particular 'unitary model' nor, except by implication, to deal with the wider 'systemic' issues, organizational and political, that are often introduced into teaching about a systems approach.

Presenting issues

The school reports to the social services that one of their 15-year-old girls is constantly missing school. When there she is always tired and though of average ability is falling well behind with her school work. The form teacher thinks that she is sexually active.

From further enquiries it is found that the girl is expected to support her mother in looking after her father and younger brother and sister. Her father has had multiple sclerosis (MS) for several years and is now increasingly disabled and confined to a wheelchair. He does not work, but spends most of the time at home, where he is said to be demanding and prone to angry outbursts.

The mother is worn down as she works part time and has also to visit her own mother who is becoming increasingly confused and frail. The grandmother receives some home care support, but this is limited because of financial constraints on the local authority.

The girl has few friends and states that she spends most of her spare time with her boyfriend, aged 17, and admits that they have started having regular sexual intercourse, though they always 'take precautions'.

Further assessment obtains information from each of the main people involved. It is important to do this in order to view the situation from as many angles as possible.

Girl Her stated concerns are:
- 'being put on at home and being treated like Cinderella';
- her younger brother and sister 'get away with doing very little' by way of chores, though they do keep their father company for some of the time;
- confused feelings regarding her boyfriend, who is putting her under pressure to have sex in exchange for giving her time and attention, which no one else does.

Mother Her stated concerns are:
- 'I feel totally overwhelmed, tired out and at the end of my tether';
- 'frustrated because I have no life of my own';
- 'guilty because I expect too much from my daughter'.

Father His stated concerns are:
- 'depressed because I am unable to be a proper father';
- 'I feel useless and unoccupied';
- 'lonely and bored'.

Brother and Sister Their stated concerns are:
- bewilderment and feeling frightened at what is happening to their dad;
- anger at their older sister because she is always 'picking on us';
- not having enough money to spend.

Worker is concerned with:
- the girl's disclosure that she is having sex under age;
- the school's negative and unhelpful attitude to the girl;
- the size of 'my workload' – very high because of staff shortages.

Assessment and action planning

In systems terms all the above statements and disclosures represent 'inputs' to the situation and will affect the process and possible outcomes. How then does an understanding of social systems help with the assessment intervention planning?

First we need to be able to identify and define the relevant social systems and their boundaries; then assess their functioning. Following this assessment it becomes possible to identify possible intervention goals and work out appropriate strategies.

Because of the interrelatedness of systems, we can take almost any starting point. For example, if we start with the girl as our initial perspective, we can think about her developmental needs and how these may or may not be being met:

- her self-concept and self-image, which may be affected by how she is dealing with her biological and physical development and social factors (personality system); here feelings about self as an individual, as a young woman, as a responsible family (female) member, and as someone who needs to find success and achievement may all need to be explored systemically.
- the influences of her family on her development, behaviour, outlook, etc. Here the family as a system clearly requires fuller investigation. In particular we would need to work out whether the stresses clearly experienced within the family constitute a current or approaching crisis and how it has coped and adjusted to its changing circumstances over a period of time.
- her social networks, which determine her relationships with adults and peers. Here there would appear to be deficits in some aspects being compensated for by the over-intense relationship with her boyfriend. Does she aspire to and can she achieve a more 'balanced' social life?
- the environmental systems that support, encourage, prevent or hinder the formation of adequate social networks and development in general (e. g. school, recreational, community and youth facilities); each needs to be mapped out and examined. Analysis of the nature and functioning of these systems will take into account issues about class, gender, race and culture and how these may all influence the situation under consideration.

From the information given it is also evident that overlaying the personal, family and social systems that provide the girl's developmental context is a fairly intense pressure system and it can be hypothesized that it is the accumulation of these pressures which account for the girl's difficulties rather than any single factor. In deciding how to intervene we are therefore presented with a number of options. Which is taken will depend on the assessment. One approach, which is not necessarily (though not excluded by it) based in systems thinking, would be to concentrate on the girl and her problems with the school. For example, we could set up a behavioural programme designed to improve school attendance and behaviour, supplemented by some individual counselling over her sexual relationships with her boyfriend (assuming there are no grounds for invoking child protection procedures).

This would seem, however, only a partial approach which ignores other influences, such as the family stresses and to what extent other situational factors operating in the school may be contributing to the difficulties. Here we might consider the school's approach to behavioural difficulties and matters of discipline generally, its approach to pastoral care, and the attitudes of individual teachers. Within a systems approach all these factors are potential targets for intervention, so that the *situational* or *contextual* factors that through assessment are found to contribute to the presenting problems can be influenced and modified. In carrying out a 'systems' assessment the 'problem' itself may therefore have to be redefined.

Examination of the effects of the girl's interactions within and between the range of systems identified suggest other possible intervention goals might be:

- to relieve the pressures operating on the family, which will take off some of the pressures on the girl and so enable her to sort out her personal difficulties more constructively;
- to encourage more positive interaction between family members and help them to feel valued and more able to support one another;
- to relieve some of the mother's objective and subjective oppression.

Achievement of any one or all of these goals could arguably assist resolution of the girl's difficulties. Time therefore needs to be spent in exploring and evaluating such possibilities as:

- obtaining more help for the grandmother, thereby reducing the pressure on the mother and consequently on the girl and other family members (an example of 'equifinality' in systems terms);
- assessing whether mother and older daughter can have more 'quality time' together, but achieving this will depend on obtaining some help for the father. Thus:
- is there support forthcoming, e. g. from the local MS society? Would he be helped by or interested in retraining or further education – or something to improve his self-worth?
- is he eligible for additional financial support that would result in more personal care being provided and therefore reduce the pressures on the primary carers?

If reductions of 'pressures' are identified as the immediate goals for the social work effort, then attention must be given to how this can be achieved most effectively. Here, the idea of creating a 'critical mass' to reduce pressures quickly in order to contain problems and make them accessible to longer term interventions is a useful one. But how can this be done given the worker's own predicament of a heavy workload and shortages within the team? The logic of the systems approach would be away from the slow drip of individual casework, where only one or two aspects of the situation can be handled at a time, to one of greater combined or team working so that a number of issues can be addressed simultaneously. The working arrangements could then be expected to be reviewed and changed as the needs of the case change. The consequences of thinking and working systemically therefore are far reaching, calling into question the whole organization of service delivery, not least at ground or 'team' level.

CONCLUSION

It is important to distinguish between a 'unitary approach', which may or not be based on systems theory, and the use of 'systems thinking' as a social work tool. One can be sceptical about unitary approaches without throwing the baby out with the bathwater and ignoring the potential value of a systems perspective in social work training and practice. Thinking systemically means thinking creatively, laterally, in patterns and looking for alternative ways of reaching common goals. Sometimes this will result in an overcoming of the familiar problem of 'we haven't got the time or the resources'. Hopefully a systems perspective will result in more strategic changes being made to social work practice, such as less reliance on individual casework, more attention to team, group and community based ways of working, and the creative use of residential care not just as residual or optional approaches, but as valid strategies.

REFERENCES

Atherton, J. S. (1989) *Interpreting Residential Life. Values To Practise*, London: Tavistock/Routledge.

Buckley, W. (1967) *Sociology and Modern Systems Theory*, New York: Prentice Hall.

Davies, M. (1977) *Support Systems in Social Work*, London: Routledge & Kegan Paul.

Davies, M. (1981) *The Essential Social Worker*, London: Heinemann Educational Books/*Community Care*.

Douglas, R. and Payne, C. (1989) *Organising for Learning*, London: National Institute for Social Work.

Goldstein, H. (1973) *Social Work Practice: A Unitary Approach*, Columbia: University of South Carolina Press.

Hearn, G. (ed.) (1968) *The General Systems Approach: Contributions Toward a Holistic Conception of Social Work*, New York: Council on Social Work Education.

Jordan, B. (1977) 'Against the unitary approach to social work', *New Society*, 2 June.

Minuchin, S. (1974) *Families and Family Therapy*, Cambridge, MA: Harvard University Press.

Payne, C. (1977) 'Residential social work', in H. Specht and A. Vickery (eds) *Integrating Social Work Methods*, London: George Allen and Unwin.

Payne, M. (1991) *Modern Social Work Theory. A Critical Introduction*, London: Macmillan.

Pincus, A. and Minahan, A. (1973) *Social Work Practice: Model and Method*, Itasca, IL: F. E. Peacock Publishers Inc.

Smale, G., Tuson, G., Cooper, M., Wardle, M. and Crosbie, D. (1988) *Community Social Work: A Paradigm for Change*, London: National Institute for Social Work.

Specht, H. and Vickery, A. (eds) (1977) *Integrating Social Work Methods*, London: George Allen and Unwin.

Thompson, N. (1991) 'Putting theory into practice. A study of practice records', *The Journal of Training and Development* 1(4): 55–60.

Triseliotis, J. (1978) 'Beyond the unitary approach', *Social Work Today*, 8 May, 20–2.

Von Bertalanffy, L., Hempel, C. G., Bass, R. E. and Jonas, H. (1951) 'General systems theory: A new approach to unity of science', *Human Biology* 1 (vi): 302–61.

Whittaker, J. K. and Garbarino, J. (1983) *Social Support Networks: Informal Helping in the Human Services*, New York: Aldine Publishing.

ADDITIONAL RESOURCES

Chris Payne talking to Malcolm Brown on 'The Systems Approach', MBA Video Productions, 1992. Distributed by Pavilion Publications, Brighton.

See also Sutton, C. (1987) *A Handbook of Research for the Helping Professions*, Part 1, 'Principles and concepts of working within the human social system', London: Routledge & Kegan Paul.

2 Task-centred work

Mark Doel

The task-centred model has its beginnings in social work practice and research. It has clear links with systems and learning theories, but as a 'home-grown' social work method of practice it is relatively unusual. Task-centred work is a systematic framework with a growing research pedigree which helps people with the practicalities of *how to do it*.

We introduce this chapter with the background to task-centred social work, followed by a detailed summary of the task-centred method, including responses to some of the difficulties encountered at different stages of the work; finally, we review the scope for task-centred practice.

BACKGROUND

The success of the task-centred approach is based on the simple idea that small successes build confidence and self-esteem, and that people are more likely to achieve these successes if they are working towards something they have chosen to do. The task-centred worker helps people to make choices about what they want to do. Central to this idea is the belief that, by and large, people are capable of reasoning and that they are the best people to make these choices.

The core values of task-centred practice are partnership and empowerment, though over-use is in danger of devaluing these terms. A partnership is two or more people working co-operatively with a common purpose; it is unlikely to be an equal partnership, in the sense that powers, roles and responsibilities are different, but a true partnership is open about these differences and seeks to redress them as much as possible. The task-centred partnership respects the fact that clients are the best authority on their problems.

'The principles of task-centred [practice] have much potential for empowering clients', writes Bandana Ahmad (1990: 51). This potential comes from the upfront way in which task-centred work addresses power and oppression. It is a method which builds on people's strengths rather than analysing their defects, providing help rather than treatment. Perhaps the most empowering aspect of task-centred work is the fact that there is no mystique about the way it works; its success depends on people understanding the processes of the work, so that they feel worked *with* and not worked *on*.

The impact of task-centred work is 'local', in that it focuses on the way structural problems such as poverty and oppression affect individuals, families or groups. This does not mean that problems are located in individuals, nor does it exclude a broadbrush understanding. It emphasizes that decisions about what to *do* are local, and this is more empowering than passively waiting to see what 'they' are going to do about it.

The Reid and Shyne study, *Brief and Extended Casework* (1969), was the twinkle in the task-centred eye, but it is perhaps not well known that the researchers – for once – did not find what they expected. They did not set out to show that brief casework would be more effective; rather they expected to confirm the conventional wisdom at the time, that brief casework would be less effective than extended casework. In fact, they found that there was no significant difference between the two. The brief casework in the Reid and Shyne study had been, literally, extended casework cut off early. Reid and Epstein (1972) went on to develop a model of social work practice which made a positive virtue of shorter time limits. They developed a systematic model with the notion of *tasks* as something central to a process of helping people with problems of living. This was the task-centred model of practice, which was further refined (Reid and Epstein 1978; Epstein 1988) and adapted to the British setting, most recently by Doel and Marsh (1992).

SEQUENCES IN TASK-CENTRED WORK

A practice method is a way of working which is systematic, both as a whole and in its different parts, so that one task-centred practitioner can recognize the work of another. However, the system should not feel like a steam-roller to the client, and the worker must adapt the method in response to different people. In practice, the sequences of task-centred work will not be as linear as they are presented on paper below. Using the tide as a metaphor, the worker's responses to the crests and troughs of the client's immediate thoughts and feelings are a part of the general tidal progress of the work, not an impediment to it.

There are three basic sequences in task-centred work, sandwiched by a period of preparation and evaluation.

Preparation

Before the first sequence in task-centred social work, there is a preparatory stage. Sometimes called the mandate for intervention, this is the point where the social worker finds out why any work should or could be done. The mandate is a shorthand way of saying 'what justifies social work at this time, in this situation?'. (For a discussion of different kinds of mandate, see Marsh and Fisher 1992: 21–4.) If this question is not considered carefully, it loosens the authority of any work which takes place and adds to confusion about what the purpose of the work is. A weak foundation for the rest of the work.

The mandate for the work might be clear: a direct request from a person voluntarily seeking help, or intervention authorized by a legal mandate. Frequently, it is less clear: one person has requested help on behalf of somebody else, who may not welcome the help, or there is a surveillance role not yet backed by the law. In these circumstances, the social worker must keep the question 'what justifies my work?' under regular review with the potential clients.

When the mandate for the work has been established clearly, each person understands the basis for the work and its purpose, and the rest of the work has a better chance of success. Ultimately, if there is no mandate, there is no work.

The first sequence: exploring problems

The first sequence of task-centred work focuses on what is wrong. What are the client's concerns and are there any additional concerns which the worker or other people in the client's life identify? Each sequence in task-centred work is, itself, broken into smaller sequences. Exploring problems is an umbrella for a number of different activities (see below), all of which are designed to help the client and the worker to understand the nature and the scope of these concerns.

Problem scanning

The first stage in exploring problems is to encourage people to discuss the range of their difficulties in a broad sense. At this point the worker is helping the client to give an overall picture of the kinds of difficulties which are being experienced. The worker's main skill is *eliciting*, so clients are encouraged to express their concerns freely. Topics might include material difficulties (such as accommodation, debts, fuel disconnection), or concerns about relationships (such as unhappiness in a marriage, problems caring for a child, feeling depressed). Nothing is excluded at this stage, not even topics which really do not seem to be any concern of social work. Few details are sought, and no solutions are offered; most of the worker's statements are aimed at scanning the range of concerns, each in turn, and communicating interest and support, with no attempt to evaluate these. It has parallels with the brain-storming technique used to help people in groups to think widely and creatively (sometimes referred to as 'blue sky' ideas). The client and social worker together list the topics they want to discuss, rather like getting an agenda together.

Problem scanning: some difficulties and responses

The client is too upset to be able to move from problem to problem
People need space to express feelings and emotions before they can feel free to think systematically. Sometimes it can take a few contacts before the client can get to this point.

The client dwells in detail on a particular problem
Workers need to explain the purpose of the problem scan; they should suggest moving on to another area, while reassuring the client that they will return to this particular topic.

The client discloses just one concern
It is intrusive to 'fish for problems' if there is only one concern which the client has, or chooses to mention. It is always possible to come back to this scanning stage a little later, giving people time to reflect on any other concerns.

The worker identifies a problem which the client does not mention
Part of the worker's explanation of the task-centred method is a commitment to honesty about sharing points of view. Workers should always be open about any concerns which they think are important to the work. Unless these additional problems put another person at risk, they should carry no more weight than the ones identified by the client.

The client identifies the worker (or the agency) as a problem
If the client's problem is the fact that the agency is on their back, this needs to be openly acknowledged. Further explanations at this point are invariably defensive and repetitive. For now, it is enough to register that this is an area of concern for the client, to be detailed later.

Problem details

Once the client and the worker have a sketch map of their concerns, it is time to look at each of them in more detail. The worker needs to be explicit about this change, so that the client can appreciate the different rhythm. The worker's main skill is *investigation*, carefully teasing out details in respect of each problem area, using open-ended questions to help the client be specific: what? who? when? where? why? how? (see *5W+H* in Priestley *et al.* 1978: 27). Answers to these questions help to put the problem into perspective. The map of problems develops from a two-dimensional sketch into a three-dimensional relief.

'For example...' is another useful prompt to help people to shape something which has felt general into something which is more definite. This careful scrutiny is supportive in the way that other methods might rely on minimal encouragers (head nods, mmmm's, etc.) or the offer of solutions. Careful listening, detailed questioning and focused interest help people feel they are being taken seriously.

Problem details: some difficulties and responses

Many concerns have been identified

It is tiring to investigate a lot of problems in close detail, so it is better to devise a 'short list' of no more than six before getting specific about each of them.

The problem changes shape when the details are described

Detailed discussion casts new light on the problem and this may challenge existing definitions of it. Ironically, a problem may shrink when it is put under the microscope, or unfold as a number of different problems. These transformations help to make the situation clearer.

The client finds it hard to answer specific questions

Thinking in generalities is easier than specifics, and the client might need some practice in answering detailed questions. The client needs to know why it is important to focus on particulars and to be prompted to think of a specific example to illustrate each problem. Any persistent difficulty in doing this should be discussed together, because of the implications for further work.

The client introduces new general topics at this stage

A thorough problem scan reduces the chances of new topics being introduced at this second stage, but if they do arise they should be listened to. However, if this is a recurring pattern, the worker should reflect on this with the client, because the success of the work relies on an ability to keep some focus.

It is hard to keep track of the details

A lot of information can accumulate during the first sequence of task-centred work. It helps to make a visual summary of what is being said, usually by writing things down briefly at frequent intervals. The client's own phrases, noted in a way that is visible to client and worker, act as a memo for them both (flip-chart paper is ideal). The headings record the topics from the problem scan, and the details from this second stage provide script. A clear statement of each problem should be recorded.

When clients have difficulties with literacy, or English is not the first language, or when the client has a visual impairment, the worker needs to develop other creative ways of providing this summary (for example, cartoons, graphics and other kinds of drawings, or brief tape-recorded summaries).

Problem priorities

The same focus which has been brought to each problem now helps people to rank these problems and to choose which one or two (three at most) to work on. This choice is a matter of judgement: the client's judgement in consultation with the worker. It does not rely on any single factor, but a balance of many considerations:

1 the urgency of the problem;
2 the consequences of not alleviating the problem;
3 the chances of success at alleviating the problem;
4 the ability of the worker and agency to help with the problem;
5 the motivation of the client to work on the problem;
6 the support which the client will receive from other people; and
7 the specific nature of the problem.

The importance of each factor will vary from one person to another and from problem to problem. Sometimes it is best to go with the client's gut feeling, which will already have been influenced by the detailed discussion of each problem.

Problem priorities: possible difficulties and responses

The client chooses a problem which is not the worker's priority
    In most circumstances the worker should go ahead with the client's priority. The worker should be frank from the beginning of contact about any problem which *has* to be included in the priority list. Workers may use a legal sanction to impose their own priorities, though the notion of a partnership between client and worker is inevitably weakened. Sometimes it is possible to agree a *quid pro quo*, where the worker and client agree to each of their priorities being included (for example, a priority problem

which the worker identifies around the client's care of a child and a priority problem which the client identifies as the agency's interference).

The second sequence: agreeing a goal and a time limit

There is a distinct change of gear between the first and second sequences. Whereas 'what is wrong?' is the theme of problem exploration, 'what is wanted?' is the theme of agreeing a goal.

We all have personal goals in life. These may be ambitious or modest, well publicized or secret, relentlessly pursued or fancifully dreamed of. They may be immediate and short term or they may stretch before us over the years. Task-centred social work builds on the research about what helps people to reach these goals. This sense of accomplishment is important to us all, but especially significant for people who have experienced discrimination, disappointment and lack of achievement.

What does the client want, in relation to the problem which has been chosen as a priority? Sometimes the client's goal may be the chosen problem turned on its head. For instance, the problem is stated: 'I'm unhappy about the way me and my daughter aren't getting on; for example, the last three times I've been to see her it ended up in a battle of words' and the goal might be: 'I want to get on better with my daughter; for example, I want to be able to get together with her once a week and not have a big argument.'

The goal should be related to the problem, but it may be indirect. For instance, the problem is stated: 'I feel lonely and isolated in this big house; for example, nobody has called to see me for the last ten days.' The goal might be: 'I want to have regular contact with other people my own age; specifically, I want to move home.'

We can see the importance of an example, because it highlights the various ways the goal could be achieved. For instance, by rephrasing the goal to: 'I want to move home so that I have regular contact with other people my own age', it is possible to see how one goal (moving home) might be seen as the stepping stone to another (getting contact with others). Options need to be explored to make sure the client feels this is the best stepping stone. This is why it is so important not to offer solutions too early in the work.

There are three key factors which the task-centred worker considers when helping people to state 'a want'. The first, and perhaps the most important, is that the goal *really* is what they want. People feel less motivated to do any work to achieve a goal which they accept reluctantly.

The second factor is practicality. What are the likely obstacles and constraints and is it feasible for the client to achieve the goal? The answer to the question, 'how much is this goal within the client's control?' will help to gauge the likelihood of success. Goals which are aimed at changing other people are less practical than ones which concern the client's own behaviour.

A third factor is the desirability of the goal. Does the worker feel that it is right to help the client achieve this goal? The client's goal might run counter to agency policy or affect the work which is going on with another member of the client's family. The worker may fear that the client's goal would cause serious harm. In these cases, the worker cannot agree to help the client to achieve the goal.

These three factors should be discussed with people in relation to possible goals, so that they can make an informed choice.

The final step in this sequence is deciding a time limit. The length of the time limit is based on the judgement of the client and the worker about how long it is likely to take to achieve the goal. A very specific goal under the client's control is likely to take less time than an ambitious goal where there are many obstacles to manage. Time limits for goals which depend on many outside factors are harder to calculate than goals where progress is more predictable. The time limit is a yardstick to mark progress towards the goal, so that people know *when* to take stock to find out if they have been successful. It is both carrot and stick to motivate the client and the worker to achieve the goal. An approaching deadline often provides the necessary shove to completion.

The likely frequency of contact between the worker and the client needs to be noted. A time limit of three months might include a weekly contact of about an hour, or daily contact for the first week, followed by fortnightly contact. A *service contract* lets people know when they will have contact with the worker and it paces the time between the beginning and the end of the agreement for task-centred work.

The chosen problem, the agreed goal and the time limit should be written clearly, with a copy for each person involved in the work. This *written agreement* between the worker and the client anchors the task-centred work, providing a brief, explicit statement of each person's commitment to the work.

Goals and time limits: some difficulties and responses

The goal is to prevent a deterioration rather than achieve a change

An elderly person might request help from the social services to stay at home. The time limit is indefinite and the goal is to keep what the client already has – independence – with the problem being a possible loss of this independence. A time limit is important as a chance to review maintenance rather than progress.

The goal involves other people

Most goals concern other people to some extent, but some goals are better reframed (for example, *'I want him to stop making me upset'* reframed as *'I want to stop getting upset when he comes home late'*). Reframing is only desirable if people truly accept it, and understand the reasoning behind it. Otherwise, is it possible to include the other people in the agreement? If not, the feasibility of the goal might be in doubt.

The client has a goal which, although desirable, the worker does not think is feasible

Task-centred social work should not be used as a stick to demonstrate to people that they are wrong. The success of the work depends on the value of positive, not negative reinforcement. The task-centred worker should convey this kind of attitude: 'To be frank, I think what you want to do isn't likely to work out, for the reasons we've discussed, but I can see you're keen to press ahead and I really hope you can achieve it. Despite my doubts, I'll do all I can to help you.' In many cases the worker will be pleasantly surprised. However, if it is unsuccessful, the worker should help the client get the best out of it and learn from the experience.

The third sequence: tasks

The journey from agreeing the goal to achieving it is measured in small steps called tasks. These are the pieces of work done by the client and the worker in order to help the client achieve the goal, which – in turn – is designed to alleviate the problem. Tasks are the rungs of a ladder which begins with the present problem and reaches to the future goal. Tasks are discussed each time the worker and client get together; first, reviewing tasks which have already been done and then developing tasks for the next stage.

Developing tasks

The factors which help to decide whether a goal is likely to be successful apply to tasks, too. *Motivation* to complete a task is enhanced if people understand why it is likely to help them to achieve the goal. The task must be *feasible*, so that the chances of success are great and it should be *desirable*. Some tasks may be repeated from one session to another; some tasks will be done by the worker and others by the client; some tasks might be reciprocal, 'I'll do this, if you'll do that.' Some tasks are best completed in the session itself (for example, rehearsing how to deal with a neighbour who is making racist remarks) and others will be done between sessions, perhaps putting into practice what has been done in the session.

The term *task* gives a false impression of physical activity, yet mental and verbal tasks are just as useful as activity tasks. The worker's main asset in this stage is *creativity*, to encourage as much variety in the tasks as possible and to harness people's strengths and interests so that the tasks tap into their abilities.

Reviewing tasks

In each session the worker and the client review all the tasks which were agreed the previous time. The first question for each task is, *was it done and if so, how successfully?* There should be positive encouragement for successful tasks, with some discussion about how easy or difficult the task was. Tasks which were unsuccessful or only partially completed need to be analysed carefully, looking at obstacles, how they were dealt with and what can be learnt from this. Often, more is learnt from unsuccessful tasks than from successful ones, so it is important not to lose this opportunity, either by attributing blame or by glossing over difficulties in a mistaken attempt to minimize the lack of success.

Tasks: some difficulties and responses

The client's motivation flags and tasks do not get done
 Sharing an observation like this helps to check if the client's interest in achieving the goal has diminished, or if something else is distracting. If it is more than a temporary distraction, or the nature of the original problem has changed, the worker and the client need to decide whether the goal needs modifying.

Progress towards the goal is buffeted off course
 Task-centred work can have quite an impact on even the most disrupted lives, but the difficulties of breaking a pattern of crisis and chaos should not be underestimated. The task-centred sequence can take place alongside other forms of work, such as crisis intervention. In extreme circumstances the worker and client might work solely on sessional tasks, moving to day-to-day tasks before attempting to build these into any more ambitious sequence of work.

The goal is achieved well ahead of time
 If this pattern recurs in the task-centred worker's practice, it may indicate that goals are being confused with tasks. A goal is something which the client would find difficult to achieve without the worker's help and usually takes many steps before it can be attained. For example, to arrange home care once a week is likely to be a worker-task rather than a client-goal, unless home care is unusually complex to achieve locally. A

goal consists of a number of tasks, where the completion of each task builds towards the achievement of the goal.

Ending the work

In task-centred social work the ending has been decided at the time of the written agreement, towards the beginning of the work. This does not always mean that contact between the social worker and the client will end; a resident will continue to see a key worker, a probationer may continue to see a probation officer. The ending refers to the period of the agreement when the client has reached the agreed goal.

The ending is a time for evaluation. Has the client achieved what they wanted? With the benefit of hindsight, was the problem selected at the beginning of the work the one which the client did want help with? The client's part in achieving the goal should be emphasized, to continue the process of empowerment.

Finally, the client's views of the task-centred way of working are canvassed. This is also a chance to rehearse the sequences of task-centred work with clients, so that they can use them independently. After all, problem solving is an everyday activity and task-centred practice is just one particularly systematic approach.

Ending the work: some difficulties and responses

The client does not want to end the work

The reasons for a person's reluctance to end the work will emerge if the ending has been prepared, by asking questions such as 'how do you think you will get on when our work is finished?'. The worker should address the specific concerns: for example, a fear that it will be difficult to get access to services again, or the loss of other gains from the work (attention, company, etc.).

The goal is not successfully achieved

If extra time is needed to achieve the goal, the time limit can be extended, but the work should not be lengthened if this only serves to prolong the agony. The likely success or otherwise of the goal is apparent before the end of the work, so it can be anticipated and the obstacles discussed. It is unusual not to have made some progress towards the goal, but in all cases it is important to focus on what can be learned rather than who can be blamed.

TASK-CENTRED WORK: LIMITS AND HORIZONS

Task-centred social work has been used with people of different ages from different cultures, with individuals, families and groups, and with a wide variety of problems (Doel and Marsh 1992: 118–22). Often characterized as a method to be used with practical problems, it is true that it is very *practical*. However, it is an approach which can be used with emotional problems just as effectively as with material ones.

Like all approaches to social work, task-centred work has its limits. In particular, it depends on a person's ability to make links between actions and consequences, and to understand the pattern of work which makes up the task-centred whole. Everybody's ability to reason fluctuates with their mood, but some people have severe difficulties in making these links, perhaps because of a mental illness or the onset of dementia. In these circumstances, it may not be possible to build the kind of partnership necessary for task-centred work; in effect, it is often a carer who becomes the client and the task-centred work takes place with this person.

Some people are unwilling clients of social work agencies, and not in the mood to enter a partnership with the worker. (See Rooney 1988, for work with 'involuntary clients.') However, the clarity of the task-centred approach helps workers and clients to know the exact nature of the disagreements, and to find out if there are any areas of mutual agreement. The task-centred worker looks for opportunities to start or extend the sense of partnership, even when the chances are slim. For example, there are opportunities for task-centred work with people on probation, even when they may prefer not to have contact with the service (Goldberg *et al.* 1984).

Task-centred practice is difficult to establish if the agency does not provide support. The professional culture of the agency may be unsympathetic to this approach, and the profile of the agency's workload might not fit the task-centred pattern, which is characterized by 'short, fat' interventions rather than 'long, thin' ones. There are many misunderstandings about task-centred social work (Doel and Marsh 1992: 91–102), not least that 'we do all that already' (Marsh and Fisher 1992: 48), and these can close people's minds to task-centred work without really understanding what it is about. Finally, heavy workloads may prevent the extra effort needed to experiment with a different method of practice.

Despite these limitations, task-centred work is well fitted to meet many of the needs of people who use social work. It is in sympathy with the growing assertiveness of user groups and their dissatisfaction with professions and bureaucracies which, for too long, have acted as if they knew what was best for the people who used their services. It is a method which empowers not only the users of the service but also the practitioners, because it provides a clear framework of accountability for their actions and an opportunity to get systematic feedback about their work – a rare commodity in social work.

In a decade which has seen the social work task increasingly defined outside the profession, the need for a well researched, 'home-grown' model of work, which is popular with the people who use it, is stronger than ever.

REFERENCES

For a full guide to the task-centred literature see Doel, M., and Marsh, P., *Task-Centred Social Work* (1992: 118–22).

Ahmad, B. (1990) *Black Perspectives in Social Work*, Birmingham: Ventura.

Doel, M. and Marsh, P. (1992) *Task-Centred Social Work*, Aldershot: Ashgate.

Epstein, L. (1988) *Helping People: The Task-centred Approach*, 2nd edn, Columbus, Ohio: C. E. Merrill.

Goldberg, E. M., Stanley, S. J. with Kenrick, J. (1984) 'Task-centred casework in a probation setting', in E. M. Goldberg, J. Gibbons and I. Sinclair (eds) *Problems, Tasks and Outcomes: The Evaluation of Task-Centred Casework in Three Settings*, National Institute Social Work Library, #47, London: George Allen and Unwin.

Marsh, P. and Fisher, M. (1992) *Good Intentions: Developing Partnership in Social Services*, York: Joseph Rowntree/*Community Care*.

Priestley, P., McGuire, J., Flegg, D., Hemsley, V. and Welham, D. (1978) *Social Skills and Personal Problem Solving: A Handbook of Methods*, London: Tavistock.

Reid, W. J. and Epstein, L. (1972) *Task-Centred Casework*, New York: Columbia University Press.

Reid, W. J. and Epstein, L. 1978) *The Task-Centred System*, New York: Columbia University Press.

Reid, W. J. and Shyne, A. W. (1969) *Brief and Extended Casework*, New York: Columbia University Press.

Rooney, R. H. (1988) 'Socialization strategies for involuntary clients', *Social Casework* 69, March, 131–40.

3 Groupwork in Britain

Allan Brown

The essence of groupwork is the benefit which can come from being together with several other people who share something in common with yourself. This shared experience may not necessarily be something that is causing concern, but in the social work context it usually is. There are many thousands of different kinds of organized groups, with much variation in aims and format, but what they nearly all have in common is interaction between people who are 'in the same boat'.

Two particular episodes in my own life which caused me much pain and anxiety illustrate this phenomenon: one was a serious illness, and the other a period of considerable emotional distress. Both times I had some support from friends and family, but on each occasion the opportunity to meet with others in a similar situation was a crucial factor in helping me to cope. When I was seriously ill there were no organized groups for people with my condition, but a few of us who attended together for treatment created our own informal group in which we were able to support each other and share anxieties and useful information about our condition and treatment. When I faced emotional turmoil, the most important support I received, both one-to-one and in organized groups, was from others who were going through or had been through a similar experience. If readers examine their own personal experiences, whether of oppression, ill health, disability, life-cycle changes, loss, or family difficulties, and then recall where they found or are finding the most help, I would expect others who have been 'in the same boat' to figure prominently.

Many groups are informal and many form spontaneously into self-help groups; others are organized and have one or more people who are called the leader or facilitator, and who undertake the role as part of their paid employment. This chapter will be mainly concerned with groups which have a measure of organization and some type of designated leader or facilitator, but many of the points made apply to all types of groups.

Groupwork is based on certain core values which are central to the method. Groups can be a source of empowerment in which people are not dependent on experts, but where they find self-esteem through being a helper of others, as well as a receiver of help; and where, for example, they can discover the collective strength to redress social oppression and take action for change. In organizational terms, groups are a 'horizontal' democratic source of peer influence and collective responsibility, by contrast with the bureaucratic 'vertical' line-management structure which is based on the concept of individual responsibility and accountability. It is not perhaps surprising, therefore, that strong effective groups, whether of agency staff or service users, are sometimes viewed with less than unqualified enthusiasm by agency managers!

Historically groupwork has strong roots in several different traditions. One of these is the settlement movement and its more recent development into youth and community work. This tradition has always been concerned with mobilizing group solidarity to combat social disadvantage and initiate social action. Another is group psychotherapy, with its emphasis on 'treatment' and the psychology of feelings, emotions and interpersonal relationships. More recent offshoots of this approach are the humanistic group therapies like gestalt, transactional analysis and psychodrama. Another tradition is seen in the self-help movement. Alcoholics Anonymous, or AA, pioneered the self-help 'leaderless' type of group which is now available for many different kinds of condition and need. Self-help groups are currently particularly strong in Scandinavia and elsewhere on continental Europe, taking over some of the territory previously served by professionally led groups (for an interesting analysis of the tensions between professional workers and self-help groups see Habermann 1990). Then there is the role of some groups in the statutory context which – although it is not always admitted openly – act as a form of social control, designed to change socially unacceptable forms of behaviour, often using behavioural or cognitive methods. Finally, in the last ten years we have seen the growth in number and prominence of groups whose primary aim is the empowerment of those sections of the population who because of their sex, class, race, disability or sexual orientation experience oppression and discrimination from those holding most of the power, whether personally or institutionally.

Mainstream social groupwork draws on all of these strands of influence, encompassing psychological and social perspectives, emphasizing the centrality of mutual aid, and laying great importance on group process and the influence of the group members themselves on what takes places in the group. It is possible to identify a number of features which are common to all groupwork groups whatever their context, purpose, clientele or methodology:

- every group has one or more purposes, whether or not these are clearly stated and agreed;
- several people will be interacting together, verbally and non-verbally;
- group members share something in common which has brought them to the same group;
- each member has the opportunity to be a helper as well as a 'helped';
- each member will be influenced by, and will influence, other members;
- what happens in the group will be significantly affected by its size and composition;
- groups change over time (not necessarily in a linear way, but some change always occurs – see below);
- issues of power and control will be an important factor in the life of the group, whether or not acknowledged explicitly;
- issues of closeness and intimacy will affect group life and individual members' behaviour;
- a group is a social microcosm which will reproduce those social attitudes, power relations and forms of discrimination – for example sexism and racism – which are prevalent in the wider society, unless active steps are taken to counteract them;
- all groups take place in a context – agency/community/socio-political – which will be very influential on group life.

Some of these group characteristics make it clear that groups can exert considerable pressure and influence on their membership – for better or for worse. If abused, this potency can be a source of pain and ethical concern: if used responsibly and with skill, it can be a source of real empowerment and positive change in people's lives. Thus while there are few who attack the whole idea and concept of groupwork, there are many who have strong views on the types of groupwork which are and are not acceptable. In many groups the members are very vulnerable, and the leaders are in a very powerful position. This is one reason for the growing attraction of group models in which the membership have control over what their group does and how it does it. However that in itself does not necessarily avoid the risk of abuse, because group members themselves can be very hurtful and controlling of other group members, as sometimes happens in self-help groups free of any professional input. One safeguard, whatever the group model, is to establish clear ground rules about how group members treat each other, together with agreed ways of responding to any breaches which may occur.

THE SCOPE AND POTENTIAL OF GROUPWORK

Having acknowledged that groupwork carries potential dangers as well as many positive features, the wide scope and potential of this method of working can be illustrated by listing some of the main kinds of needs which can benefit from a skillful and sensitive group approach.

Physical health   Many groups are set up to try and meet the needs of people who either have health problems themselves, or are carers/close relatives of those affected. For example, groups for people with AIDS (Getzel and Mahony 1989); groups for parents of children with terminal illnesses (Engebrigtsen and Heap 1988); groups for older people in residential care whose health is deteriorating (Lewis 1992); groups for people with cancer (Daste 1989).

Emotional and mental health   Examples include groups for adolescent female child sexual abuse victims (Craig 1990); for those with agoraphobia (Rose 1990); those suffering from schizophrenia (Randall and Walker 1988); and those who have been ground down by the sheer pressures of living in intolerable circumstances of poverty and disadvantage (Breton 1991; Lee 1991).

'Linked-fate'   Whitaker (1985) coined this term to describe groups for family members who have special needs because they are closely related to others with special needs: for example, siblings of children with disabilities (Badger 1988); children of divorced parents (Regan and Young 1990); non-abusing mothers of abused children (Masson and Erooga 1990).

Empowerment   A range of groups are now becoming available for women (Butler and Wintram 1991; Donnelly 1986; Mistry 1989), black people (Mullender 1988; Lee 1991), and others who experience social discrimination and oppression. One of the main purposes of these groups is to create a group climate in which members can rediscover their own value and self-esteem, and become empowered both to improve their own lives and, collectively, to take action for social change (Garvin and Reed 1983; Davis and Proctor 1989; Mistry and Brown 1991; Brown 1992, chapter 6).

Behaviour change   Statutory agencies have found that groups can be a particularly effective way of influencing individual behaviours that cause hurt to others, for example, offending behaviour groups (McGuire and Priestley 1985), groups for perpetrators of sexual abuse (Erooga, Clark and Bentley 1990), alcohol education groups (Baldwin 1990). Cognitive methods (Ross, Fabiano and Ross 1986) which attempt to change members' thought patterns are now used quite extensively as the method of choice for this type of group.

Life transitions and their consequences Transitions involving major adjustments whether as a 'natural' part of the life-cycle like starting employment, having a baby, or retiring; or due to some form of state intervention, for example, leaving local authority care or prison (Fisher and Watkins, in press); or some disruption in family life, for example divorce; or the effects of political crises such as becoming a refugee (Tribe and Shackman 1989).

Educational This category includes life and social skills groups (Priestley *et al.* 1979), literacy groups, outdoor activities, youth groups.

Self-directed and social action groups This type of group offers members full responsibility and control over what happens, both for themselves and the group as a whole (Mullender and Ward 1991). Group goals are usually external to the group with the aim of bringing about change in the members' social environment.

Group living In daily life in residential and day centres, people participate in a whole range of groups and groupings. What happens in any particular group or gathering affects, and is affected by, what is happening elsewhere. This requires the groupworker to have particular kinds of skills and understanding (see Brown and Clough 1989, for accounts of groupwork in different centres, and a conceptual framework for thinking about working with groups in these settings).

KEY FACTORS IN GROUPWORK PRACTICE

There are key factors which anyone planning or participating in a group needs to take account of. These are:

Thorough preparation The importance of preparing properly cannot be overstated. With new groups this may include advocacy in the agency to establish the support and resources (people and things) necessary for providing a facilitative environment for the group. It also involves everyone being clear what the group is for, what it will do, when it will meet, what the ground rules will be, and so on.

Group size and composition Whether the group is self-help or worker led, is concerned with social control or social action, the size and composition will have a profound effect on what happens. An ideal size is quite small, say five to seven people, when there is a fairly natural tendency to gel. As it gets larger so more attention needs to be given to group organization to make sure that everyone is fully included in what happens, and to reduce the often unhelpful effects of splintering and subgrouping. The guide to composition is to seek both a basic sameness – or homogeneity – in what members have joined for, providing a source of support, *and* a good variety – or heterogeneity – of types of people and personalities to provide fertile conditions for stimulation and change.

It is important to try not to have 'singletons' in groups if at all possible. This means not having just one man or woman or one black or white person or one younger or older person in a group, because this can put a lot of pressure on that individual to 'represent' their kind, in the process constraining their own freedom to be themselves and to gain the maximum personal benefit. Control over group composition is not, of course, always possible or even desirable – there is the issue of freedom of choice for the lone female, black or older person who may say they do not see any problem, particularly if no other choice is available – which means that if there are singleton members the group must do everything possible to ensure that person is not 'labelled'.

The worker(s)   The three crucial questions are: how many workers are needed, who the worker(s) will be, and what his or her or their role(s) will be in the group. On the first point, does the group really need to have more than one worker? Bearing in mind that workers are a scarce resource, there need to be good reasons for having more than one, and these are likely to include the type of group, the needs and abilities of the group members, the size of group, the level of experience and skills of available workers, and so on (for a fuller discussion of these and other co-working issues see Hodge 1985, Preston-Shoot 1987, and Brown 1992: 77–88). If there are to be two co-workers – as is common in Britain – a good working relationship is essential which means checking out compatibility and capacity to work together effectively. In male/female and black/white pairings, strategies need to be worked out to ensure that the patterns in the wider society of men and white people holding most of the power will not be replicated in the group (Mistry and Brown 1991).

The third issue of the role/s of the worker/s in the group is probably the most significant of all as it will have a profound effect on the group process and the role of members. In some models the workers are unashamedly the leaders from beginning to end; in others they start in the 'central role' but gradually devolve responsibility and control to the group members as the group progresses; and in others the understanding is that the group will be self-directed from the beginning with the worker in the role of facilitator or consultant rather than leader (as in the early stages of some self-help groups).

Group purpose Whatever the type of group, members need to be clear what they are there for. All groups need to be aware of the three levels of the individual, the group and the external environment, but the relative emphasis on each of these varies greatly depending on the type of group. The crucial thing is to have a shared understanding of purpose between all who are involved.

Open and closed groups Every group, once it is established, has to decide whether its membership is closed or whether new members can join; and if it is open what the rules, if any, are about when and how people join and leave. Some open groups, like 'drop-ins', fluctuate considerably in membership from meeting to meeting, others have much more gradual and carefully planned changes (see Henry 1988).

Group agreement and ground rules Joining a group is a big step to take, particularly for people who are not used to being in organized groups. The potential member needs to know whether the group is likely to be a safe non-threatening place. Ground rules on vital issues like confidentiality, equal space and opportunity, no violence, anti-racism, anti-sexism, anti-disablism, and attendance expectations, are no guarantee about what will and will not happen in the group, but at least give the potential member some idea of the underpinning values. They also provide a clear basis for workers or members to intervene if unacceptable behaviour occurs.

Group programme What will the group do? How much will be decided in advance? and who will decide? These are all crucial questions, and misunderstandings often occur: 'I was told this was a discussion group and now I am being expected to do role-play and drama.' Again, there needs to be full discussion about programme and method, and a shared understanding about what has been decided.

Task and process Group task is what the group is there for, its purpose. Group process is about the life of the group and what happens between its members. Some groups are much more task orientated than others, but process is always important, because how members are feeling about each other, the worker/s and the group as a whole will have a major impact on the degree of success in achieving the task. Skilled workers and members are those who are able to strike the right balance in which the process of the group is harnessed to enhance task achievement.

Stages of group development As mentioned earlier, every group changes over time. The 'linear' or straight line approach suggests that groups go through a succession of predictable stages, starting with group formation, then a period of struggle for role and position, then a coming together as the group gels, then a period of 'maturity' when the group is most productive, and finally a period of ending and disengagement (Tuckman's model of forming, storming, norming, performing and ending, 1965). This pattern has some validity for some groups, but real life is much more complicated(!) with many groups showing periodic circular or spiralling tendencies. Perhaps most significant of all is the stage – by no means reached by all groups – at which the group membership takes ownership of the group, and 'their' group becomes 'our' group.

Consultation, recording and evaluation   Is consultation and/or supervision needed and available? Will group life and progress be recorded? And how will the group be evaluated? These are all important matters to be thought about before the group gets under way (see Brown 1992, chapter 7; and Preston-Shoot's article on evaluation, 1988).

GROUPWORK PRACTICE EXAMPLES

Two contrasting group examples illustrate good practice and the potential of groupwork to be an effective and empowering source of help to people in need.

The first example (Mistry 1989) illustrates, among other things, how proactive workers can take group initiatives which not only result in a new and empowering group service, but which can also have the wider impact of influencing agency policy and practice. This author describes the innovation and development of a women offenders group, based on feminist principles, in the context of a quite traditional probation setting in which all the senior managers at that time were male and white. The spur to set up the group came from the not unusual situation of women offenders being marginalized in groups and groupwork approaches which were designed for the male majority of offenders. There was either no available group provision for females or they had to join highly structured predominantly male groups not at all suited in structure, content or style to their needs as female offenders.

Against this 'male' background, Mistry and one or two women colleagues launched a pilot group for black and white female offenders, with a feminist perspective which viewed their offending behaviour 'within their socio-economic position in a patriarchal society'. The group sought to promote women taking control of their own lives and used group methods which were responsive to the women's own concerns rather than fitting them into structures and norms determined by the group leaders. Initially the workers faced considerable resistance both from colleagues (mostly male) and from senior management who initially viewed all-female groups with some suspicion. The pilot was followed by a group which continued for several years and gradually gained agency approval and support, not least because it was successful in reducing levels of re-offending by the women.

The group was based on voluntary contracted attendance, and the underlying philosophy was one in which decisions and arrangements were negotiated with group members who had a real sense of shared ownership of the group with the women probation officers who were the official leaders. For the women, it was 'their' group, not something alien being imposed on them by others. The programme included a wide range of topics, many proposed by the group members themselves, for example childcare, poverty, sexuality, racism, sexism, the criminal justice system, offending and domestic violence. A 'move-on' second stage self-help group was formed, indicating how important meeting in a group had become to the women, although, as often happens, funding problems led eventually to its closure.

The second example concerns adolescent girls who have been sexually abused (Craig 1990). An age-related group approach is often the preferred method of working with children and adolescents who have been abused, because of the strength and support that can come from peer sharing and exchange at a time of great vulnerability and lack of trust in adults. This type of groupwork is highly skilled and should not be undertaken without special training and good consultation and support for the workers, in this case staff from the NSPCC and other agencies in Rochdale.

This group had two 'simple but important general aims', the first 'to provide a safe forum where victims could explore and resolve the feelings of isolation, shame and stigmatisation which result from the abuse' and the second to help the participants accept that they were not in any way responsible for the abuse – they were the 'victim' and someone else was the 'offender' – and to begin 'the journey from victim to survivor'. Meeting with other 14 to 18-year-old girls who shared similar experiences and feelings, under the skilled guidance of two female workers, and in a safe environment with clear ground rules, provided the opportunity to work at incredibly painful and difficult matters. The group used a variety of methods including not only discussion but also body image work, exercises, opening and closing 'rituals', for example sharing 'how we are' at the beginning of each meeting, guided fantasies, confronting a cushion with things which it has not been possible to say directly to the perpetrator, and so on.

In this group, as in many groups, a clear structure provided security for the first few meetings, after which the group became more spontaneous with the agenda being determined increasingly by what was uppermost for members at any particular meeting. One illustration of what could only be possible in a group setting was the sharing of experience of, and rehearsing for, the traumatic experience of being a witness in court proceedings and having to confront the perpetrator. The author stresses the importance of evaluating groupwork, and in this group it was done both subjectively by the use of self and peer evaluation, and rather more objectively by asking referring professionals to complete assessment forms both before and after the group experience. Craig concludes that there are often 'observable and tangible' short-term positive gains from their groups, but adds an important word of caution about the need for longer term follow-up to determine whether there are lasting benefits. This caveat applies to all groupwork: snapshot evaluations give only a partial and often temporary view of the impact of any group or group session on an individual.

THE CURRENT STATE OF GROUPWORK

In conclusion I shall now consider a few issues surrounding the current state of groupwork in Britain (for developments in North America see the journal *Social Work in Groups*; and in continental Europe, Heap, 1989 and 1992).

Social work in Britain in the early 1990s is experiencing a time of major change due to the combined effects of radical new legislation (the Children Act 1989, the National Health Service and Community Care Act 1990, and the Criminal Justice Act 1991); a quite hostile political climate committed to a reduced function for statutory social work; and a chronic shortage of resources relative to expanding need – for example, arising from demographic changes and higher expectations of quality of service. One consequence of these developments is the not-so-gradual transfer of some mainstream social welfare provision, particularly in day and residential care, to the voluntary and private sectors. Another is the squeezing out of any provision in the statutory sector of social work activity other than that required by statute.

The consequence of this for groupwork in social services departments and probation areas is quite far-reaching. In the former, where groupwork has always been quite patchy, it appears to be contracting other than in day and residential settings, and in areas of statutory responsibility, for example child protection. But even where groups are supported in principle, the combination of reduced resources, preoccupation with procedures to the detriment of therapeutic work, and continuing resistance by some senior managers to 'horizontal' methods like groupwork which confuse line-management accountability, has meant that offering groups and particularly those involving creative imaginative work, takes considerable determination and tenacity. It is true that a few social services departments, particularly in the London area, demonstrate a commitment to groupwork by appointing senior groupwork consultants, but this is the exception rather than the norm. We know rather more about the situation in probation because of a quite recent national survey (Caddick 1991) into the extent and range of groups being run. The returns, based on the situation in 1989, show, first, that groupwork was being practised quite extensively in all probation settings, and, second, that there was a fairly equal incidence of groups concerned with the modification of offending behaviour and those 'whose objectives lean more towards providing developmental or enabling experiences for the members'. However, an analysis of group aims made it clear that most groups – the exception being some groups for female offenders – concentrated on offenders as individuals (the 'remedial' model) rather than on the causative factors in their socio-cultural context. Moreover, since this survey of 1989 data, the parameters have changed quite dramatically with the implementation in 1992 of the new punishment-orientated Criminal Justice Act. It now seems likely that the trend towards the control imperative in groupwork with offenders will accelerate (see Brown and Caddick, in press).

An encouraging counterpoint to these trends in statutory agencies is the growing emphasis on groupwork based on empowerment, particularly of women, black people and other oppressed groups. Two strands can be detected in this development. One is the impetus coming from a feminist groupwork perspective both within and outside statutory agencies (see Mistry 1989 and Butler and Wintram 1991), and the other is the development of the 'self-directed' model of groupwork (Mullender and Ward 1991). The latter approach, which operationalizes empowerment as a method as well as a value, is based on the notion that, guided by the worker as facilitator, members create their own agendas, predominantly to seek change outside themselves in the social context in which they live.

It will be interesting to see to what extent this countervailing emphasis on empowerment – to which all managers are likely to subscribe at least in theory – can be sustained in the statutory climate outlined above and elsewhere in this book. The associated concern is that we shall have groups which are increasingly task-orientated in emphasis, with decreasing attention being paid to process, which I consider to be the life-blood of groupwork. If we fail to accord importance to *how* people work together in groups we are reducing groupwork – at least in statutory agencies – to a rather sterile exercise in which group members receive packaged group programmes of limited usefulness, making no real impact on them as unique individuals often caught up in oppressive social conditions of poverty.

In some of the traditional larger voluntary agencies, for example Family Service Units and Barnados, creative groupwork continues to thrive and be innovative, though there too, the decline in adequate resourcing is having its impact on social workers and the range of services that can be offered. It is not yet clear how much scope there will be for groupwork in the expanding private and independent sectors, but with finance-led policies and a shortage of trained staff it is not easy to be optimistic.

Finally, in reviewing groupwork in Europe, past, present and future, Heap (1992) points to two interesting trends in mainland Europe, particularly in Scandinavia. The first is the reality that much of the groupwork that is now being undertaken is being done by professionals other than social workers, for example nurses; and, second, the accelerating trend towards the widespread use of self-help groups. Both of these developments present a challenge to groupworkers in the social work tradition, not to try to protect or rebuild their crumbling empire, but rather to be selective in concentrating on the kind of groupwork which they do best – groupwork in which both group process and the enormous resources of the group membership are viewed as central in all that happens.

REFERENCES

Badger, A. (1988) 'A group for children with physical disabilities', *Groupwork* 1(3).
Baldwin, S. (ed.) (1990) *Alcohol Education and Offenders*, London: Batsford.
Breton, M. (1991) 'Towards a model of social groupwork practice with marginalised populations', *Groupwork* 4(1).
Brown, A. (1992) *Groupwork*, 3rd edn, Aldershot: Avebury.
Brown, A. and Caddick, B. (eds) (in press) *Groupwork with Offenders*, London: Whiting & Birch.
Brown, A. and Clough, R. (eds) (1989) *Groups and Groupings: Life and Work in Day and Residential Centres*, London: Tavistick/Routledge.
Butler, S. and Wintram, C. (1991) *Feminist Groupwork*, London: Sage.
Caddick, B. (1991) 'Using groups in working with offenders: a survey of groupwork in the probation services in England & Wales', *Groupwork* 4(3).
Craig, E. (1990) 'Starting the journey: enhancing the therapeutic elements of groupwork for adolescent female child sexual abuse victims', *Groupwork* 3(2).
Daste, B. (1989) 'Designing cancer groups for maximum effectiveness', *Groupwork* 2(1).
Davis, L. and Proctor, E. (1989) *Race, Gender and Class: Guidelines for Families, Individuals and Groups*, New Jersey: Prentice-Hall.
Donnelly, A. (1986) *Feminist Social Work with a Women's Group*, Social Work Monographs 41, Norwich: University of East Anglia.
Engebrigtsen, G. E. and Heap, K. (1988) 'Short-term groupwork in the treatment of chronic sorrow', *Groupwork* 1(3).
Erooga, M., Clark, P. and Bentley, M. (1990) 'Protection, control, treatment: groupwork with child sexual abuse perpetrators', *Groupwork* 3(2).
Fisher, K. and Watkins, L. (in press) 'Inside groupwork', in A. Brown and B. Caddick (eds) *Groupwork with Offenders*, London: Whiting & Birch.
Garvin, C. and Reed, B. (eds) (1983) *Groupwork with Women/Groupwork with Men*. Special issue of *Social Work With Groups* 6(3/4), New York: Haworth Press.

Getzel, G. and Mahony, K. (1989) 'Confronting human finitude: groupwork with people with AIDS', *Groupwork* 2(2).

Habermann, U. (1990) 'Self-help groups: a minefield for professionals', *Groupwork* 3(3).

Heap, K. (ed.) (1989) *Groupwork in Europe. Groupwork* special issue 2(3).

Heap, K. (1992) 'The European groupwork scene', *Groupwork* 5(1).

Henry, M. (1988) 'Revisiting open groups', *Groupwork* 1(3).

Hodge, J. (1985) *Planning for Co-leadership*, Grapevine, 43 Fern Ave., Newcastle upon Tyne, NE2 2QU.

Lee, J. (1991) 'Empowerment through mutual aid groups', *Groupwork* 4(1).

Lewis, G. (1992) 'Groupwork in a residential home for older people', *Groupwork* 5(1).

McGuire, J. and Priestley, P. (1985) *Offending Behaviour; Skills and Strategems for Going Straight*, London: Batsford.

Masson, H. and Erooga, M. (1990) 'The forgotten parent: groupwork with mothers of sexually abused children', *Groupwork* 3(2).

Mistry, T. (1989) 'Establishing a feminist model of groupwork in the probation service', *Groupwork* 2(2).

Mistry, T. and Brown, A. (1991) 'Black/white co-working', *Groupwork* 4(2).

Mullender, A. (1988) 'Groupwork as the method of choice with black children in white foster homes', *Groupwork* 1(2).

Mullender, A. and Ward, D. (1991) *Self-directed Groupwork: Users Take Action for Empowerment*, London: Whiting & Birch.

Preston-Shoot, M. (1987) *Effective Groupwork*, London: Macmillan.

Preston-Shoot, M. (1988) 'A model for evaluating groupwork', *Groupwork* 1(2).

Priestley, P., McGuire, J., Flegg, D., Hemsley, V. and Welham, D. (1979) *Social Skills and Personal Problem Solving*, London: Tavistock.

Randall, L. and Walker, W. (1988) 'Supporting voices: groupwork with people suffering from schizophrenia', *Groupwork* 1(1).

Regan, S. and Young, J. (1990) 'Siblings in groups: children of separated/divorced parents', *Groupwork* 3(1).

Rose, S. (1990) 'Group expression: a method of treating agoraphobia', *Social Work with Groups* 13(1).

Ross, R. R., Fabiano, E. and Ross, R. D. (1986) *Reasoning and Rehabilitation: A Handbook for Teaching Cognitive Skills*, Ottawa: Cognitive Centre.

Tribe, R. and Shackman, J. (1989) 'A way forward: a group for refugee women', *Groupwork* 2(2).

Tuckman, B. W. (1965) 'Developmental sequence in small groups', *Psychological Bulletin* 63(6); 384–99.

Whitaker, D. (1985) *Using Groups to Help People*, London: Routledge & Kegan Paul.

FURTHER READING

Benson, J. (1987) *Working Creatively with Groups*, London: Tavistock.

Glassman, U. and Kates, L. (1990) *Group Work: A Humanistic Approach*, London: Sage.

Groupwork, published in Britain by Whiting & Birch; three issues p.a.

Heap, K. (1985) *The Practice of Social Work with Groups*, London: George Allen & Unwin.

Houston, G. (1990 edn) *The Red Book of Groups*, London: The Rochester Foundation.
Social Work with Groups, published in the USA by Howarth Press; four issues p.a.
Yalom, I. (1985 edn) *The Theory and Practice of Group Psychotherapy*, New York:
Basic Books.

Training manuals

Henderson, P. and Foster, G. (1990) *Groupwork Skills Pack*, Cambridge: National
Extension College.
Kemp, T. and Taylor, A. (1980) *The Groupwork Pack*, London: Longman.

4 A participatory approach to social work

Suzy Croft and Peter Beresford

The modern history of social work is one of constant change and attack. The role, organizational setting and philosophy of social work have all undergone change at an accelerating pace. Over the last twenty years there has been a shift from caseworker, to community social worker and now care manager; from 'specialism' to 'genericism' and back again. Social work's critics question whether it even has its own distinct body of knowledge. It is attacked by the political left for being a soft cop, by the political right for inducing dependency and by the tabloid press for the series of child care tragedies and scandals that punctuated the 1980s and early 1990s.

Social work is currently undergoing another period of drastic change. This time it's part of much broader changes in society and welfare, reflected in the move to a changed 'economy of care', the 'purchaser–provider split' and a 'contract culture'. Now the rhetoric is of more 'user-centred' services and a key idea informing this is 'user involvement'. There are many different reasons for this development, but most can be traced to dissatisfaction with the postwar welfare state. They include:

- the rise of the political right and election of Conservative governments opposed to government intervention and large-scale public welfare;
- wider public disquiet about the poor quality and unaccountability of welfare and other public services;
- the emergence of a wide range of organizations and movements of people who received and were dissatisfied with such welfare services;
- progressive welfare professionals seeking to work in more egalitarian ways;
- the emergence of pioneering initiatives providing different, more participatory services and offering new role models;
- increased interest in ideas of citizenship, civil rights and equal opportunities;
- the emergence of new philosophies like normalization and a social model of disability.

Characteristically, social work, like other welfare services, has been *provider-led*; that is to say the providers of service, including politicians, managers, academics, researchers, planners and practitioners, have shaped it, *not* the people for whom it is intended. A number of key problems are associated with such provider-led services, including institutionalization, paternalism, inadequate safeguards for the rights of service users, and abuse.

Interest in a more participatory approach to social work is not new (Beresford and Croft 1980). The 1968 Seebohm Report which led to the setting up of social services departments talked of 'citizen participation' and recommended both individual and group participation in the provision and planning of services (Seebohm 1968). Ideas of involvement and empowerment have long been high on the agendas of progressive social work practitioners. There is a hidden history of clients struggling to gain more say in social work. Community work approaches linked with social work have also placed a particular emphasis on local involvement.

But social work's track record on participation has generally been poor. Deakin and Wilmott, in their pioneering study of participation in local social services in two London boroughs, for example, found little involvement of either service users or other local people in one of them. They reported that there was evidence of constraints in developing participation at almost every level. 'Although the thinking and public statements of the [other] authority were conducive to participation, we encountered some scepticism about implementation... at policy and planning levels.' In both boroughs they concluded that 'representing the consumer voice did not seem to be a high priority for councillors at least over social services matters' (Deakin and Wilmott 1979).

Sixty per cent of users of social services departments, in a 1982 study by Sainsbury and others of clients' and social workers' perceptions in long-term social work, felt that workers had acted contrary to their own expressed wishes (Sainsbury *et al.* 1982: 21). Tyne, in his 1978 study of participation in policy making and planning by families of people with learning difficulties, reported that social services departments were often quite unprepared to let parents' groups in on the process of policy making or service planning (Tyne 1978). People with learning difficulties themselves were even less likely to be involved in social work and social services. Oliver, writing in 1983 about social work with disabled people, argued that 'there is no relationship between the needs of disabled people and the services they receive. Rather, disabled people have their needs defined and interpreted by others' (Oliver 1983: 124,130).

The Client Speaks by Mayer and Timms, published in 1970, the year the Local Authority Social Services Act set up social services departments, is remembered as the book which first offered clients' views about social work.

It revealed a massive level of misunderstanding between clients and case-workers. The authors wrote that there was 'an often Kafkaesque quality about these worker–client interactions'. But they, like their social work subject, largely ignored issues of race and gender. They reported uncritically the social worker

> ... who told one man to 'Go out more. Let the woman do the job in the home'. They excluded people from the sample who were not born in the British Isles, 'since the reactions of "non-natives" to social work are likely to be complicated by cultural differences, language problems and so forth'.
>
> (Beresford and Croft 1987: 52).

The Client Speaks was not a plea for social work to involve or listen to the voice of its clients. The authors were mainly interested in clients as another data source for researchers. There is no discussion of how consumers' views could be involved in a process of practical change. Instead *The Client Speaks* set a different trend, initiating another area of academic and professional study which came to be called 'client studies' and which was a cul de sac as far as the involvement and empowerment of social work clients were concerned (Fisher 1983). It's only more recently that ideas of involvement have extended beyond this.

While terms like user involvement and participation have now gained greater currency in social work, there is little agreement about what they mean. The history of participatory initiatives is also confused and chequered (Beresford and Croft 1992). It may therefore be helpful to begin to clarify what we mean by involvement.

When people talk about getting involved, they most often mean helping out in some way. This involvement essentially entails some kind of voluntary work. But such responsibility need not be and is usually not accompanied by any increase in the say or control that people have. Self-help initiatives sometimes bridge the gap. As Crewe and Zola said, writing about disabled people:

> Self-help groups ... have become a powerful source of mutual support, education and action among people affected by particular health concerns or disabilities.... While learning and working together, disabled people can combine their power to influence social and political decisions that affect their lives.
>
> (Crewe and Zola 1983: xiii–xiv)

As this emphasizes, the purpose of involvement, beyond voluntary action, is to bring about *change*. As we shall see later, who actually leads that change and where control over it lies may vary, but change is the unifying aim of all participatory initiatives, except of those which are deliberately obstructive or disempowering.

A wide range of arguments are now offered for increasing people's say in social work and social services. They emphasize its importance on both practical and philosophical grounds. Let's look at some of these arguments more closely.

Most people want to be involved. It's not surprising that most of us want some say in agencies and decisions which can have important effects on our lives. Two-thirds of a random sample of people we surveyed in one neighbourhood where there was a move to more community-orientated social services were in favour of service users having more say and involvement in social services (Beresford and Croft 1986: 228). This reflects other research which indicates that most people want more say in their local communities and in institutions and services which affect them (Beresford and Croft 1978). The deprivation of people who use social services has sometimes been seen as a particular problem limiting their interest in or ability to get involved, but the proportion of social service users in our sample wanting more involvement was similar to the sample overall. The desire for more involvement is also directly reflected in the growth and objectives of disability, rights and self-advocacy organizations. These include many recipients of social work services.

People have a right to be involved. Rights can be categorized in several ways. Rights which have particular relevance here are human rights, civil rights and legal rights. Social work can clearly impact on all these. Its interventions extend to the most intimate and personal aspects of our lives. It has powers to restrict people's rights and we know that on occasion it has failed to respect them. Having a say in social work is an important expression of people's rights. More specifically people now have legal entitlements to be involved. The government's stated commitment from the 1980s to 'people power' and consumer choice means that there are now legal requirements for public involvement in a wide range of public services, from health to education, housing to land use planning. The National Health Service and Community Care Act and the Children Act extend this to social work. People now have rights to redress, to comment and to be consulted about social work.

People's involvement in social work reflects the democratic ethos of our society. Many question marks may be placed over the reality of this ethos. The western tradition is also more clearly one of representative rather than participatory democracy. But there is no doubt that the idea of democracy is a powerful and guiding one in Britain and other western market economies.

It is important that social work alongside other state interventions can clearly be seen to be consistent with this. There is a growing view, strengthened by the highly publicized series of contentious social work interventions concerned with child sexual abuse in the 1980s and early 1990s, that the involvement of service users and other citizens is necessary if social work is to be a democratic activity.

Involvement increases accountability. Accountability means that individuals and organizations are not just responsive to people but *answerable* to them. People have a right to know what is happening and why and for their questions to be answered. People who seek involvement in social services are sometimes told that they already have this involvement through their elected councillors. In reply they often argue for a more direct accountability. Accountability may be direct or indirect. If it is distant or indirect; to local electors generally, rather than people using services specifically; to parents, rather than people with learning difficulties themselves, then it can seem like another expression of paternalism rather than effective accountability, with one group speaking on behalf of another. Direct accountability demands people's involvement or the involvement of *their* organizations and directly elected representatives. Increased involvement results in more effective accountability.

Participation makes more efficient and cost-effective services. The efficiency argument is currently one of the most powerful. So far there is little clear evidence of a direct link between increased 'user involvement' and enhanced economy and efficiency, but this may be due to the fact that few such studies have been carried out. It may also be that the relationship between involvement and the 'three Es' – efficiency, economy and effectiveness – is more complex and less direct than is assumed. However the idea has a strong commonsense appeal. 'Who knows better where the shoe pinches than the wearer?' Particular weight is also attached to this argument because of the emphasis commercial organizations place on market research and consumer involvement to maximize their profitability and market share. If social workers want to provide the support and services that people actually need, then involving them in the process is likely to avoid duplication and inappropriate provision, improve 'targeting' and create pressure for more effective and responsive systems of management.

Involving people accords with social work goals. This is the argument that comes closest to social work philosophy. People's involvement is important because it is consistent with the aims of social work. Ideas of enabling and supporting people's independence and self-determination have long been at the heart of social work. The British Association of Social Workers' *Code of Ethics* states that the basis of social work:

... is the recognition of the value and dignity of every human being, irrespective of origin, race, status, sex, sexual orientation, age, disability, belief or contribution to society. The profession accepts a responsibility to encourage and facilitate the self-realisation of the individual person with due regard to the interests of others.

(BASW, undated)

It is difficult to see how this could be achieved in an unequal relationship in which the 'client' has only a limited say and qualified involvement, which is located in an organizational setting over which the 'client' has no control. This seems more likely to create and perpetuate passivity and dependence.

Involving people challenges institutionalized discrimination. Arguments that social services are white, male-dominated and Eurocentric are well rehearsed and well evidenced (Hanmer and Statham 1987; Langan and Day 1992; Dominelli 1988; Hugman 1991). While the majority of both workers and service users are women, senior managers are still predominantly white men. Black people are still more likely to experience the controlling than the supportive aspects of social work and social services. Support services are often inaccessible to or inappropriate for members of black and other minority ethnic communities (Dutt 1990). A participatory approach to social work offers a direct challenge to existing patterns of discrimination and exclusion by involving service users and other local people with all their diversity of age, race, gender, class, disability and sexual orientation.

While as we have seen, strong arguments are offered for increasing people's involvement in social work, some reservations are also expressed. We want to look at two of the most important of these.

The first concerns people's *competence* to participate and it is raised in regard both to children and to adults – for example, those with learning difficulties or dementia (Stevenson 1990: 5).

Chronological age is notoriously unreliable as an indicator of children's ability to participate. Research into children's intellectual, social and emotional development increasingly suggests that they can make a contribution about how they are treated and what they want from a very early age. Different children and children of different ages may be able to participate in different ways and to different degrees, but then the same is true for adults. There is strong evidence to support greater involvement by children and young people in decision making. What it requires is particular sensitivity to how children are involved and what support they are offered (Hodgson 1993).

The rights of children are particularly vulnerable. This is an added reason to involve children, not to exclude them.

Participation is not an all or nothing activity. Instead of assuming that there will always be 'some people' who can't be involved, the responsibility should be on proving that expert skills and support are so far insufficient to enable them to. The emphasis on people's inability to participate persists among many managers and professionals. But denying people opportunities for involvement then reinforces the problem because their abilities are obscured and inhibited. Members of groups of disabled people, people with learning difficulties and older people we have spoken to, all describe a similar process:

> The initial objection to us taking part was that we hadn't got the skills. Then we got involved and spoke up and they said we... hadn't really got learning difficulties. We weren't typical of disabled people. Or they'd say someone put us up to it! They just couldn't believe we can speak for ourselves.
>
> (Beresford and Croft 1993: 18)

The second reservation about involving people who use services is raised where social workers have powers and responsibilities to *restrict* people's rights, perhaps to safeguard those of others. But interventions that restrict people's rights don't have to and *shouldn't* exclude their involvement. It is needed more than ever in such circumstances. Research is also beginning to confirm that such involvement is feasible in practice (Marsh and Fisher 1992). The question is not so much how you reconcile people's participation with restrictions on their rights, as how justice can be done if people are denied any say or involvement in such decisions. When people's rights are in question, their involvement and empowerment are essential to ensure that:

- they are kept fully informed at all stages;
- they and their representatives can put their case;
- they are fully involved in the making of the decision;
- they are fully aware of what decisions are made and why;
- they can appeal against decisions;
- they are involved in the review of decisions.

What we want to do next is start to chart the universe of a participatory approach to social work. It is a universe which is more complex and multi-faceted than may first be apparent. There are different spheres for such involvement in social work. These include people's involvement in:

- their personal dealings with agencies and services;
- running and managing agencies and services;
- planning and developing new policies and services;

- initiating and providing their own support and services.

People may be involved on an individual or collective basis, representing their own interests or as a member or representative of an organization which they collectively control. Their involvement may relate to individual or collective services. For instance, some disabled people run their own self-operated support schemes. Some have established integrated or independent living centres.

There is a wide range of areas for people's involvement in social services agencies and service provision. These include involvement in

- expenditure and budgetary control;
- staff recruitment;
- training;
- standard-setting;
- quality assurance;
- inspection;
- designing and placing contracts;
- monitoring and evaluation;
- providing services;
- designing and controlling individual support schemes.

There are now a growing number of examples in all these areas. For instance, a local health authority and social services department commissioned People First, the organization of people with learning difficulties, to carry out an evaluation of two group homes and local day services as part of their hospital closure policy (Whittaker *et al.* 1991). In the London Borough of Hammersmith, service users with HIV are members of a quality control group alongside managers, social workers and local voluntary organizations, contributing to regular quality assurance meetings and involved in setting standards (Murray 1991: 18–19). People using social services are making an increasing contribution to social work training. In 1992 the Central Council for Education and Training in Social Work organized a day conference bringing together educators and people who used social services to develop guidance for good practice in involving service users in training.

Safeguarding services users' rights is also a key part of a participatory approach to social work. This has three key components, all of which extend people's participation:

- data protection;
- effective complaints procedures;
- access to records.

A participatory approach to social work is not only concerned with the involvement of people who use services. We have always argued that *all* four key constituencies in social services – service users, carers, workers and other local people – must be involved if participation is to be empowering and not divisive. The empowerment of service users will not come through the further disempowerment of service workers. Workers need to be empowered too (Croft and Beresford 1992: 175–6). Many face-to-face workers experience similar oppressions to the people with whom they work. The involvement of workers in the development of a participatory approach to social work will help ensure that it is workable and that it is actually implemented. Three key components will support this. These are:

- workers' rights are agreed and protected;
- support is provided for staff to work in a participatory way;
- staff involvement is ensured in developing participatory provisions and practice.

At the heart of a more participatory approach to social work is a more participatory practice. We have talked to many social work practitioners and service users about what makes for a more participatory and empowering practice (Beresford and Croft 1993). Qualities they emphasize include:

- giving people a choice of service and practitioner;
- starting with a clear and agreed code of practice;
- presenting people in positive not demeaning images;
- listening to what people say;
- keeping people informed by providing full and appropriate information, interpreting and translated materials;
- using accessible and positive language;
- offering people support not direction;
- employing people with direct experience of services as service users;
- seeing the whole person in context;
- enabling reciprocity and exchange by seeing people's strengths as well as their difficulties.

Most of these may seem principles for good, rather than specifically participatory practice. Perhaps the two are one and the same thing. Such principles are certainly consistent with those goals of enabling people's independence and supporting self-determination, which as we have said are traditionally associated with social work and social services.

We identify four important dimensions to a participatory practice.

The aim of practice is to empower people – challenging oppression and discrimination rather than reflecting them and making it possible for people to take greater charge of their lives.

Practice offers people control in their personal dealings with agencies – allowing them to participate in what happens to them instead of being kept in an excluding or passive relationship. Five components of practice are usually identified:

- assessment;
- planning;
- recording;
- action;
- review.

Service users should be involved in them all: defining their own needs and having a say in planning and decision making.

Practice equips people to take power – enabling them to participate by helping them gain the confidence, self-esteem, assertiveness, expectations, knowledge and skills needed to have an effective say.

The agency in which practice is located is open to people's involvement – offering opportunities, structures and resources for a say in its working.

A participatory practice cannot be conceived of in isolation from the agency in which it is offered. A more participatory practice is unlikely to be possible without more participatory agencies. A participatory practice ideally puts people in a position to have more say and offers the first and most concrete expression of their involvement. Counselling, rights work, information giving, group and community work can all form part of a participatory practice.

An example can be given from the practice of Suzy Croft. In her work as a job-share social worker, she has learnt to value eight key components for a participatory and empowering practice:

- make no assumptions;
- recognize the different, sometimes conflicting, interests involved;
- the need for negotiation;
- support people to regain control;
- the importance of advocacy;
- validate people's own abilities and experience;
- be honest and give accurate information;
- enable choice.

Croft works in a terminal care support team, but these components are likely to be just as important in other settings. They may also offer a basis for participatory and empowering policy. Those components may be looked at more closely through the experience of one woman, Judy.

Judy was widowed four years before breast cancer was diagnosed. She had a job, lots of friends and a daughter aged 14, Sarah.

It would be easy to imagine a woman full of anxiety and fear about her future, who had seen her sister die of breast cancer four years earlier, wondering who would look after her daughter and tempting to want to talk about these with her. When I met Judy, that's not what she wanted. She wanted help with her money, applying for benefits and to get a washing machine. She refused advice from the nurse on the team about controlling the symptoms of her cancer. She wanted to be in control and we had to respect that. It wasn't until later that she wanted to talk about her feelings.

Judy's cancer didn't just raise questions about her interests. What about Sarah's? Community care often involves *competing interests*. Judy's approach of not thinking about her cancer and not planning for the future was her choice. But what might it mean for Sarah? We knew Judy wouldn't live long. It was important for Sarah to know that and for them to plan her future together. As I got to know Judy better I asked her if she'd made any plans for Sarah. She seemed prepared for my question. 'Oh, yes. We have started to think of it.'

I also needed to *negotiate* between Judy and Sarah. They had lots of arguments. Judy thought she was 'no good as a mother' because 'I can't do anything for Sarah any more.' But lots of teenage daughters do their own cooking and ironing. Sarah criticized her mother's 'weepy', irritable behaviour because she didn't know she was in pain. Judy needed to tell her she was. Judy was determined to fight and carry on 'as normal'. Sarah couldn't understand it when she couldn't keep this up. We talked about it.

Tears poured down Judy's face one day as she said: 'I feel I have no control of what's happening to me.' *Regaining control* was crucial to her. We sat down and talked about what she could do. She decided to have work sent home, have a home help and another course of chemotherapy.

As she became more ill, *advocacy* became increasingly important. She told the doctor about the uncontrolled pain in her leg and that she felt the drugs he had prescribed were making her confused. Nothing happened. I 'phoned him. He seemed surprised and a bit taken aback but agreed to rearrange her drugs. Advocacy is not the same as taking over from people, denying their abilities and patronizing them. It's about recognizing and validating *their competence and capacity* to cope. In the team we try and recognize the right of each person to face death in his or her own way.

Judy's health got worse. When I saw her I was shocked by the change

in her appearance. She asked me, 'How do you think I look?' I could have
said 'You look fine.' I said what I felt was the truth. 'You look very sad.'
She cried and told me she had asked the doctor how long she would live.
He said 'months not years'. 'Do you think I could have a remission and
live years? Does that happen to any of your patients who have the same
cancer as me?' I though Judy wanted an *honest* discussion. She was dying
and needed to be able to talk about it. I told her I had never heard of anyone
with an advanced disease like hers having a remission. There was a long
silence, then Judy said, 'I needed to know.' Then she talked about telling
Sarah she might only live a short time and said she wanted to be the one
to do that.

I found out that one of Judy's friends was very angry with me. She felt
I shouldn't have talked to Judy about dying. It had made her 'give up'. I
discussed it with her. I said I thought Judy had made an important *choice*.
She was extremely ill and was ready to accept she was dying. She needed
to talk about it and not be told 'don't talk like that', making her feel lonely
and isolated.

Judy decided she would like to go into a hospice, but she became too
ill to be moved. Three friends were with her when she died. Two weeks
later I bumped into Sarah in the entrance hall of her school as I went for
a meeting. She told me about her plans for Christmas, where she was going
to live and who would have her two cats and dog – there was an old dog
who hated other animals in her new home. She was planning a memorial
service to be held on Judy's birthday.

(Croft 1992: ii–iii)

Increasing people's say and involvement is a contentious issue. We can
expect it to generate opposition and resistance. It arouses fear and hostility
among some powerholders. The most common response people can expect
to encounter when they try and become more involved in social work and
indeed other services is that they aren't '*representative*'. Our own research
suggests that this is the objection against 'user involvement' most often
expressed by service providers (Croft and Beresford 1990: 35–7). It is
perhaps ironic that in the past, when representation in welfare mainly meant
speaking on someone else's behalf, there was little argument, but now when
people are trying to speak for *themselves*, it is becoming a much more
controversial issue. Democratically constituted disability and self-advocacy
groups can expect to have their representativeness challenged regularly.
Service users experience this as marginalizing and demeaning. Questioning
people's right to be involved on this basis can serve as a convenient excuse
for continuing to exclude them and for service providers to hang onto the
power they have.

At the same time, representation poses some real problems. There are real difficulties in the way of involving a wide range of people in any participatory initiative, particularly in a society like ours where there is not a strong culture or tradition of participation and where disability, rights and service user organizations generally don't have the resources they need to reach out to as many people as they would wish. As we have already argued, extending people's involvement in social work offers a way of challenging the institutionalized discriminations that exist in both its structures and practice. But if there isn't equal access in involvement, then that involvement will merely mirror and reinforce existing race, gender and other discriminations.

Two components appear to be essential here if people are to have a realistic chance of exerting an influence and all groups are to have equal opportunities for involvement. These are *access* and *support*. Both are necessary. Experience suggests that without support, only the most confident, well resourced and advantaged people and groups are likely to become involved. This explains the biased response that participatory initiatives have typically generated. Without access, efforts to become involved are likely to be arduous and ineffectual.

Access, in the specific context of services, includes physical accessibility, the provision of services which are appropriate for and match the particular needs of different groups, and access points providing continuing opportunities for participation within both administrative and political structures, including membership of subcommittees, planning groups, working parties and so on.

The need for *support* arises not because people lack the competence to participate in society, but because people's participation is undermined by or not part of the dominant culture or tradition. People may not know what's possible or how to get involved; may not like to ask for too much or be reluctant to complain. There are five essential elements to support. These are:

- personal development: to increase people's expectations, assertiveness, self-confidence and self-esteem;
- skill development: to build the skills they need to participate and to develop their own alternative approaches to involvement;
- practical support: to be able to take part, including information, child care, transport, meeting places, advocacy, etc. ;
- support for equal opportunities: provision for disabled people, deaf people, people with sensory impairments, without verbal communication, non-readers, people for whom English is not their first language and people with intellectual impairments;
- support for people to get together and work in groups: including administrative expenses, payment for workers, training and development costs.

Earlier we discussed the wide range of developments that have led to increased interest in a more participatory approach to social work and social services. This has been reflected in the emergence of two difference conceptions of and approaches to involvement: the *consumerist* and the *democratic* approaches. It is important to distinguish between the two. They reflect different philosophies and objectives. The first has been associated with the politics of the new right and the second with the emergence of disabled people's rights and service user organizations.

The *consumerist* approach has largely been developed by service providers. Here the aim is primarily to improve the efficiency, economy and effectiveness of services. Service users can help in this by contributing their ideas and experience to improve management and decision making. The enormously expanded interest in consultation and market research in social services is one highly visible sign of this approach.

The *democratic* approach is not service centred. It is concerned with people having more say and involvement in their lives, not just in services. It is concerned with people's empowerment, with their civil rights and equality of opportunity, and sometimes with the achievement of broader social change.

The emergence of consumerist thinking in health and welfare services has coincided with the expansion of commercial provision and a growing political emphasis on the market. Consumerism starts from the idea of buying the goods and services we want instead of making collective provision for them. Two competing meanings underpin the idea of consumerism: first, giving priority to the wants and needs of the 'consumer'; and second, conceiving of people as consumers and 'commodifying' their needs, that is to say, converting these needs into markets to be met by the creation of goods and services.

These two areas of potentially conflicting meanings – between a consumerist and a democratic approach to involvement, and between a consumerism which puts the consumer first and one which puts market consideration first – have major implications for a participatory approach to social work.

There is no doubt that currently the dominant approach to ideas of involvement in health and welfare is the consumerist, not the democratic one. At the same time concerns are growing that under the new consumerist arrangements of care, it is the requirements of the market not the needs of the consumer which are becoming paramount. Let's look at this more closely.

While the stated aim is to move from a *service* to a *needs*-led system of social work and social services, there are growing fears that the shift may actually be from a service to a *budget*-led system (Simmons 1992: vi–vii). A 1992 report of the multi-agency Policy Forum warned that community care reforms and the Children Act were facing a 'credibility gap' among service users and could founder without more resources. It uncovered evidence of a 'patchwork' of unequal provision (Harding 1992). In another report, Alvin Schorr, the distinguished American commentator, concluded that British personal social services were caught on a downward slope that would lead to their irretrievable breakdown. He pointed to the inadequacy of funding for the services, arguing for greater resources or more limited goals (Schorr 1992). A 1992 survey showed social services departments nationally making major cuts in expenditure (Hatchett 1992: 18–19).

The president of the Association of Directors of Social Services talked of 'home help services being withdrawn from some elderly people, continuing care declining in the health service, falling adaptations to people's homes and a work backlog for occupational therapists' (*Community Care* 1992: 3). This reflects the more impressionistic picture we have gained from our own contact with many practitioners, managers, carers and users of social services in different parts of the country: a picture of reduced services, increased charges and more restrictive rationing. Disability and service user organizations report a similar picture (Cervi 1991a: 5; Cervi 1991b: 2). While the Social Services Inspectorate's report *Care Management and Assessment* stated that the rationale of the government's community care reforms was 'the empowerment of users and carers' (Social Services Inspectorate 1991), in 1992 the High Court judged that residents of local authority homes for elderly people had no rights to be consulted before decisions were taken to close them (Ivory 1992: 6).

The care manager role, which is central in the new arrangements for care, similarly raises important issues for a participatory approach to social work. Two things are striking about this role. First, it places consumers in a very different relationship to goods and services from the one they are generally used to in the market place. Here the service user isn't the purchaser of service; the health or social services authority is. The service user doesn't decide what support she or he needs; the care manager does. It's a strangely paternalistic version of the exchange relationship. Second, it requires a major change in the role and tasks of social workers. The responsibilities of the care manager include assessment, co-ordinating services, creating 'care packages', negotiating between and consulting with different service suppliers, carers, service users and their organizations and controlling budgets. Many of these demand different skills from those traditionally associated with social work. Social work is not necessarily the profession which first comes to mind as having them. Significantly Sir Roy Griffiths made no reference to social workers in his influential report on the future of community care (Griffiths 1988). Already home care organizers are being recruited as care managers because of their budgetary experience.

Taken together these new arrangements, the creation of a 'care market' and the role of care manager, run the risk of combining the shortcomings of both state and market systems, with services provided according to cash not need, and needs defined by professionals not service users.

In this chapter we have tried to describe a participatory approach to social work for which there now is growing support among service workers, service users and carers. We have also set this in the context of current policy developments. This raises two broader questions. First, what kind of role is there for social work in the new mixed economy of care? Second, is the current consumerist policy consistent with a participatory approach to social work? It will be some time before we know the answers to these questions. So far the indications are not encouraging.

REFERENCES

Beresford, P. and Croft, S. (1978) *A Say in the Future: People, Planning and Meeting Social Need*, London: Battersea Community Action.

Beresford, P. and Croft, S. (1980) *Community Control of Social Services Departments*, London: Battersea Community Action.

Beresford, P. and Croft, S. (1986) *Whole Welfare: Private Care or Public Services?*, Brighton: Lewis Cohen Urban Studies Centre.

Beresford, P. and Croft, S. (1987) 'Are we really listening?', in T. Philpot (ed.) *On Second Thoughts: Reassessments of the Literature of Social Work*, Sutton: Reed Business Publishing/*Community Care*.

Beresford, P. and Croft, S. (1992) 'The politics of participation', *Critical Social Policy* 35.

Beresford, P. and Croft, S. (1993) *Citizen Involvement: A Practical Guide for Change*, London: Macmillan.

British Association of Social Workers *Code of Ethics for Social Work* (undated), Birmingham.

Cervi, B. (1991a) 'Disabled people incensed by home help reforms', *Community Care*, 9 May.

Cervi, B. (1991b) 'Disability groups unite to fight home help cuts', *Community Care*, 11 July.

Community Care (1992), 23 January, news.

Crewe, N. M. and Zola, I. K. (1983) *Independent Living for Physically Disabled People*, London: Jossey-Bass.

Croft, S. and Beresford, P. (1990) *From Paternalism to Participation: Involving People in Social Services*, London: Joseph Rowntree Foundation/Open Services Project.

Croft, S. and Beresford, P. (1992) 'User views', *Changes: International Journal of Psychology and Psychotherapy* 0(2), June.

Croft, S. (1992) 'Empowerment in action', Inside Supplement, 'Involving service users', *Community Care*, 26 March.

Deakin, R. and Willmott, P. (1979) *Participation in Local Social Services: An Exploratory Study*, Studies in Participation, London: Personal Social Services Council.

Dominelli, L. (1988) *Anti-Racist Social Work*, London: Macmillan.

Dutt, R. (1990) 'Community care and black people', Community Care Supplement, *NCVO News*, London: National Council for Voluntary Organisations, January/February.

Fisher, M. (ed.) (1983) *Speaking of Clients*, Sheffield: Community Care/Joint Unit for Social Services Research, Sheffield University.

Griffiths, Sir Roy (1988) *Community Care: Agenda for Action*, London: Department of Health.

Hanmer, J. and Statham, D. (1987) *Women And Social Work*, London: Macmillan.

Harding, T. (1992), *Great Expectations... And Spending On Social Services*, Policy Forum Paper No. 1, London: National Institute for Social Work.

Hatchett, W. (1992) 'Charting the swing of the axe', *Community Care*, 21 May.

Hodgson, D. (1993) *Children's Participation in Social Work Planning – Practical Pointers from the Experiences of Young People and Social Workers*, London: National Children's Bureau.

Hugman, R. (1991) *Power in Caring Professions*, London: Macmillan.

Ivory, M. (1992) 'Home closure: An open and shut case?', News Focus, *Community Care*, 16 July.

Langan, M. and Day, L. (1992) *Women, Oppression and Social Work*, Issues in Anti-Discriminatory Practice, London: Longman.

Marsh, P. and Fisher, M. (1992) *Good Intentions: Developing Partnership in Social Services*, York: Joseph Rowntree Foundation/*Community Care*.

Mayer, J. E. and Timms, N. (1970) *The Client Speaks*, London: Routledge & Kegan Paul.

Murray, N. (1991) 'Their own boss', *Social Work Today*, 17 October.

Oliver, M. (1983) *Social Work with Disabled People*, London: Macmillan.

Sainsbury, E., Nixon, S. and Phillips, D. (1982) *Social Work in Focus: Clients' and Social Workers' Perceptions in Long-term Social Work*, London: Routledge.

Schorr, A. L. (1992) *The Personal Social Services: An Outside View*, York: Joseph Rowntree Foundation.

Seebohm Committee *Report of the Committee on Local Authority and Allied Social Services* (1968) Cmnd 3703, London: HMSO

Simmons, D. (1992) 'Needs versus cash', Inside Supplement, 'Involving service users', *Community Care*, 26 March.

Social Services Inspectorate (1991) *Care Management and Assessment, Summary of Practice Guidance; Managers' Guide; Practitioners' Guide*, Department of Health, London: HMSO.

Stevenson, O. (1990) 'Empowerment and opportunity', in P. Stevenson, S. Croft, P. Beresford and D. N. Jones, *Empowerment and Opportunity*, Birmingham: British Association of Social Workers.

Tyne, A. (1978) *Participation by Families of Mentally Handicapped People in Policy Making and Planning*, London: Personal Social Services Council.

Whittaker, A., Gardner, S. and Kershaw, W. (1991) *Service Evaluation by People with Learning Difficulties*, London: King's Fund Centre.

FURTHER READING

Beresford, P. and Croft, S. (1993), *Citizen Involvement: A Practical Guide for Change*, London: Macmillan.

Croft, S. and Beresford, P. (1990) *From Paternalism to Participation: Involving*

People in Social Services, London: Joseph Rowntree Foundation/Open Services Project.

Croft, S. and Beresford, P. (1993) *Getting Involved: A Practical Manual*, London: Joseph Rowntree Foundation/Open Services Project.

Dowson, S. (1991) *Moving to the Dance: Or Service Culture and Community Care*, London: Values Into Action.

'Involving service users' (1992) Inside Supplement, *Community Care*, 26 March.

Jordan, B. (1990) *Social Work in an Unjust Society*, London: Harvester/Wheatsheaf.

Morris, J. (1991) *Pride Against Prejudice: Transforming Attitudes to Disability*, London: Women's Press.

Oliver, M. (1990) *The Politics of Disablement*, London: Macmillan.

Stanton, A. (1989) *Invitation to Self-Management*, London: Dab Hand Press.

Thompson, C. (ed.) (1991) *Changing the Balance: Power and People Who Use Services*, Community Care Project, London: National Council for Voluntary Organisations.

5 Community work

Marjorie Mayo

Community work has its own history within the development of social work in Britain. But community work has been taking place in a range of other settings too, and community workers have been applying their community work skills to professional work around community health, community education, housing and planning, community employment and youth and community work (to name some of the better known examples) both within statutory agencies, and within the voluntary and informal sectors. Given this diversity of community work settings, the definition of 'community work' takes on particular importance. What are the common strands within these different areas of practice? And how can social workers use community work methods themselves, and relate to other community workers most effectively, whether these community workers are employed within social work agencies, or within other relevant agencies, concerned with community welfare more broadly?

In a recent review of current realities and contemporary trends in community work, Butcher has argued that there are a wealth of different definitions of community work, but that 'in an effort to be comprehensive, they tend to be rather lengthy, (Butcher 1992:144). In summary, these definitions have considered community work as being concerned to enable people to develop collective responses to shared needs, whether these needs relate directly to the concerns of social service departments, such as community care or childcare needs, or whether these community needs effectively require responses from one or more different agencies, crossing departmental and sectoral boundaries. Twelvetrees has defined community work 'at its simplest, as being the process of assisting ordinary people to improve their own communities by undertaking collective action' (Twelvetrees 1991: 1). And community work has been, by definition, particularly concerned with the needs of those who have been disadvantaged or oppressed, whether through poverty, or through discrimination on the basis of race, class, gender, sexuality, age or disability.

Even the term 'community' itself has been problematic, covering as it does a range of different meanings. Within these different usages, however, sociologists have identified two major approaches to defining 'community': community in terms of the people who live in a common geographical area (such as a social services patch), the community of locality; and community in terms of common interests (such as ethnic origin, or disability, or shared concerns about caring for a child with special needs) (Bulmer 1987:28). Both types of usages are relevant and important for community work.

Forms of community work developed in Britain over a century ago from the settlement houses, starting with Oxford House (founded in 1883) and Toynbee Hall (1885) which were established as local centres for the delivery of social work services and other neighbourhood activities, including community education. Other strands in the history of British community work include the development of the community association movement in the interwar period, and the development of tenants' associations (see Clarke 1990).

In the 1960s and early 1970s, community work in Britain has been described in terms of its diversity and its dynamic growth (Community Work Group 1973:9). As Hadley has argued, at this time 'the achievements of the post-war welfare legislation were critically reassessed' in the light of continuing economic and social deprivation, and 'new kinds of collective intervention were explored'.... 'Further, it was argued that the paternalistic style of invervention that had characterised state-run services had discouraged popular interest and involvement, and that more participative methods of managing services should be encouraged' (Hadley *et al.* 1987:2). The government itself launched a national experiment, the Community Development Project, in 1969, drawing upon experiences elsewhere, including experiences of community work in the United States. Debates on the restructuring of social work also included a growing 'community focus' (Loney 1983:22). The Seebohm Committee (Seebohm 1968:147) stressed that 'we see our proposals not simply in terms of organisation but as embodying a wider conception of social service, directed to the well-being of the whole community and not only of social casualties, and seeing the community it serves as the basis of its authority, resources and effectiveness'. The report's recommendations included support for community work within area social services teams, together with recommendations that social services should provide support for the voluntary sector, and for consumer participation more generally, within the framework of preventive approaches to community social welfare.

A decade on, in the early 1980s, it was clear that these aspects of the Seebohm Report had not been effectively implemented. But the issues were still alive and the importance of community social work was a major theme in the Barclay Report (1982:198) which argued that 'the personal social services must develop a close working partnership with citizens focusing more closely on the community and its strengths', recognizing that 'the bulk of social care in England and Wales is provided, not by the statutory or voluntary social services agencies, but by ordinary people (acting as individuals or as members of spontaneously formed groups), who may be linked into informal caring networks in their communities' (pp.199–200). The Barclay working party was influenced by the work of Hadley and others on neighbourhood or patch based community social work, work which Hadley and others continued to develop in the 1980s (e. g. Hadley *et al.* 1987). The development of community social work continued to be problematic in practice, however, although there were a number of local authorities which did move in this direction, just as there were local authorities and local authority organizations which made significant commitments to the promotion of community work and community development more generally, in relation to specific services such as housing, recreation and community education, as well as at corporate level (AMA 1989).

By the end of the 1980s, there was renewed interest in community work in the context of debates around the mixed economy of welfare. The type of welfare pluralism which was advocated in the Griffiths Report on community care, for instance, would entail closer collaboration between statutory and voluntary agencies, with greater emphasis upon the role of informal, community based care, self-help, mutual aid, and user involvement (Griffiths 1988). Bamford has highlighted the continuity here between the concerns of Seebohm, Barclay and Griffiths (Bamford 1990). Whilst the NHS and Community Care Act 1990 has been the key in reviving potential interest in community work, similar themes have emerged in other contemporary initiatives, including the Children Act 1989 with its recognition of the role of preventive work in the community in, for example, family centres. There have been important developments in the use of community work approaches to child care, in practice, both in family centres, and in other aspects of preventive child care, including residential care (Gibbons and Thorpe 1989; Harlesden Community Project 1979; Holman, 1983). More generally, too, the Citizen's Charter (1991) has raised issues around citizens' rights and the quality and appropriateness of public services, although these rights have been posed in terms of individuals, rather than in terms of communities. (User participation and user rights are central issues in community work, and are considered, in their own right, in chapter 4.)

By now it will have become only too clear that community work has taken on a range of meanings, in the widely differing contexts of the settlements of the late nineteenth century, through to government projects, local authority programmes and community based initiatives in the informal sector, in the late twentieth century. It has been associated with policies from both right and left. Twelvetrees has categorized the different approaches to community work in terms of 'professional' community work, in contrast with 'radical' community work, the latter drawing upon neo-Marxist and feminist analyses of society. He defines the 'professional' approach in terms of professional concerns to promote self-help, and to improve the effectiveness and appropriateness of service delivery, within the wider framework of existing social relations. Alternatively, the 'radical' approach emphasizes the potential contribution of community work to shifting the framework of existing social relations, empowering the powerless to question the causes of their deprivation, and to challenge the sources of their oppression, with a focus upon anti-racist and anti-sexist work (Twelvetrees 1991). Having set out these distinctions, however, Twelvetrees has also recognized that these have been greatly oversimplified.

There is a further difficulty with Twelvetrees' use of these terms to describe the different approaches to community work. The designation of one approach as 'professional' could be taken to imply that the other 'radical' approach was in some way 'unprofessional' (although this is not an argument which is put forward by Twelvetrees himself). In fact, of course, professional values, knowledge and skills are essential for community work practice, regardless of the theoretical perspectives of particular practitioners. It might therefore be less confusing to categorize Twelvetrees' 'professional' approach as the 'technicist' approach, meaning an approach which focuses upon the application of community work techniques, regardless of wider debates about values and underlying social relations.

In contrast, the 'radical' approach focuses upon the potential relationship between community work and wider strategies to promote the empowerment of those who have been disadvantaged through the social construction of race, class and gender relations. But the term 'radical' has itself been used in different ways in recent years, being applied to fundamental challenges from the 'radical' right, as well as from the 'radical' left. As an alternative, the term 'transformational' has the advantage of implying a practice which is geared towards empowerment, development and liberation. The term has been applied in both first and third world contexts, emphasizing the importance of democratic methods as well as objectives in community development (see Hope and Timmel 1984).

In practice, of course, whatever their concept of community work, community workers have to operate within the constraints of their particular situations, both in terms of the interests of their employers, and in terms of the interests of their client communities. And studies of what community workers actually do have shown that they tend to spend their time supporting community groups working on immediate issues, with relatively modest reformist goals (Barr 1991; Butcher 1992:152). Given the immediacy of the massive practical problems and unmet needs within the type of communities which have professional community work support, it would perhaps be more surprising if this were not the case. But it is important to recognize that community work has been and continues to be developed within the wider framework of different and competing political agendas. There are right-wing versions of community enabling, for example, geared towards the promotion of self-help, to rolling back the state, and substituting for public responsibility in service provision, just as there are radical versions of community enabling, with more focus upon democratic participation and community empowerment, for social transformation.

Whatever their varying theoretical perspectives, community workers share a range of community work methods, together with a range of knowledge and skills. The study group report *Community Work and Social Change* (Gulbenkian Foundation 1969) identified three main levels of community work:

- grass roots or neighbourhood work (working with local individuals, families and community groups);
- local agency and inter-agency work (working with local umbrella organizations, federations and other local-authority wide organizations, together with local statutory and voluntary organizations);
- regional and national community planning work (for example, working on economic development issues, planning and environmental issues which span wider than the local boundaries).

In practice, of course, as the subsequent study group report concluded, 'the interrelation between these three levels of community work is continuous' (Community Work Group 1973:12). Community work within social service departments clearly involves both neighbourhood work and local agency and inter-agency work, for example, typically with a focus upon service development, for one or more client groups (community care provisions being based upon precisely such a mix). Whilst agency and inter-agency work, and social and community planning work are central to community work, however, a number of authors have drawn attention to some of the dangers of work at these levels. In particular, social planning work can lead community workers to substitute themselves for the communities which they are committed to supporting and enabling (Twelvetrees 1991). This point relates, in turn, to the question of different community work approaches, directive and non-directive methods.

Community work methods have been defined in terms of two ends of the directive/non-directive continuum. Non-directive approaches were characterized by Batten in terms of where decision and action lie with the members of the group themselves. The characteristics are self-determination, a process where the group identifies its own needs, makes its own plans and works largely by self-help to their realisation. The community worker is an enabler in this process, not the director or manager.

In contrast, directive methods are

> where the main decisions are taken by the official or leader or council and programmes and policies are worked out on this basis. Imposition rather than self-determination is the characteristic and active participation may be limited to a small committee or inner official group.
>
> (Batten 1967, quoted in *Current Issues*, 1973:13).

Batten himself was a strong advocate of the non-directive method on grounds of principle and practice believing that directive methods tended to be counterproductive in the long run.

Since then, the non-directive method has itself been criticized on a number of grounds, including the view that, in an unequal society, community workers who are totally non-directive, without being prepared to raise issues of inequality and oppression, end up by reinforcing the status quo (Filkin and Naish 1982:36–47). It has, in fact, become widely accepted that community workers do have a professional responsibility to challenge discrimination and oppression, even when they are committed to the non-directive method. So, for example, if a community group were to discriminate, either directly or indirectly, against black or ethnic minority residents, the community worker who works with that group would have an overriding responsibility to challenge that racism, regardless of the community work method which was being employed. Many local authorities now include equal opportunities provisions, both in terms of their own policies, and in terms of their arrangements for grant aid to the voluntary sector, including community groups.

While the non-directive method has been subject to criticisms and review since Batten developed it in the 1960s, there are features which may still be relevant and useful in the 1990s. For example, it has been argued that the implementation of the NHS and Community Care Act 1990 may lead to pressures on community workers to deliver, in terms of care in the community. But ultimately, community workers may have to argue that community groups, like individuals and families, have the right to self-determination. If they choose to provide community care services, that has to be their decision, rather than the decision of the community worker who is employed to support the development of community care in the neighbourhood. But community groups cannot be directed to provide care services. This is not in any case realistic, any more than it is realistic to assume that community workers can set up carers' groups, for instance, if not actively supported by the carers concerned. Nor could, or should, individuals or community groups be directed to substitute for cutbacks in necessary jobs and services such as domiciliary services (Twelvetrees 1991) (although there have been proposals to enforce volunteering as a condition of receiving benefits in workfare-type schemes, for example). And community workers may have to argue that as professionals committed to equal opportunities, they should never direct women to provide care in the community in ways which undermine women's rights to equal opportunities, whether in terms of opportunities for paid employment, or in terms of social relations, in the family and in the community.

Community workers need a range of knowledge and skills in order to practise effectively. Typically, community workers' tasks involve some combinations of the following:

* making contact with individuals, groups and organizations;
* developing a community profile, assessing community resources and needs;
* developing a strategic analysis, and planning aims, objectives and targets;
* facilitating the establishment of groups;
* facilitating the maintenance and effective development of groups;
* working productively with conflict, within and between groups and organizations;
* collaborating and negotiating with other agencies and professions;
* relating effectively to policy making and implementation, including local politicians;
* communicating orally and in writing, with individuals, groups and organizations;
* working with individuals, including counselling;
* managing resources, including staff time and budgets;
* supporting groups and organizations in obtaining resources, e. g. grant applications;
* monitoring and evaluating progress, and the most effective use of resources;
* withdrawing from groups, and/or facilitating the effective ending of groups;
* developing, monitoring and evaluating equal opportunities strategies.

This is by no means an exhaustive list. But community workers should be competent to carry out all of these tasks if they are to function effectively, in a variety of settings. In order to do this, community workers need to have knowledge of the relevant policy areas, including the appropriate legislation. So, for example, they need a background understanding of social policy and welfare rights, together with more specific knowledge in relation to the issues which are central to their particular post, such as relevant housing and planning legislation for community workers in housing departments, for instance, or child care and community care legislation for community workers in social service departments. In addition, community workers need to have knowledge and understanding of the socio-economic and political backgrounds of the areas in which they are to work, including knowledge and understanding of political structures, and of relevant organizations and resources in the statutory, voluntary and community sectors. And they need to have knowledge and understanding of equal opportunities policies and practice, so that they can apply these effectively in every aspect of their work.

In relation to specific practice skills, community workers need to have confidence in their skills in the following key areas:

* engagement;
* assessment, including needs assessment;
* research;
* groupwork;
* negotiating;
* communication;
* counselling;
* management, including time management and financial management;
* resourcing, including grant application;
* recording and report writing;
* monitoring and evaluation.

While this list may sound formidable, in practice many if not most of these skills are transferable to and from other areas of practice. In fact, many of these established areas of community work knowledge and skills are precisely the skills which social workers may most need to develop, in the changing context of social work in the 1990s (Bamford 1990). And many of these areas of knowledge and skills are also shared by unpaid community workers and activists. This follows from the starting point that 'there is no monopoly on the term community work, nor should there be' (Twelvetrees 1991:13). Paid community workers have responsibility for valuing and supporting the knowledge and skills of unpaid community activists, working in partnership with them. And paid community workers should be ensuring that unpaid community workers and activists have maximum access to further education and training. Current developments in training, such as the work on National Vocational Qualifications, through the Federation of Community Work Training Groups, have been geared to maximize the value given to experiential learning, and to maximize community access to further education, training and professional qualifications.

The Barton Project, Oxford, provides examples of a wide range of community work at different levels, linked into education and training provision for professional social and community workers as well as for volunteers and activists. The project was established in 1974 in a peripheral postwar housing estate which had been identified as one of the city's high-stress areas. Starting as a joint initiative by the local authority and the university, the project now works closely with both city and county councils, with local community organizations, with voluntary agencies such as Oxford MIND and the Children's Society, and with a number of social and community work training courses. The project includes community work on social work related issues such as community care, with a community care worker employed by social services working from the project. Information and advice services are provided to local residents and groups, covering welfare benefits, housing and debt problems on a neighbourhood basis as part of the project's anti-poverty strategy. Specialist welfare rights support and training is provided to social services staff, and other agencies on a county-wide basis. In this way community social work is linked into wider preventive work and community development. The project undertakes research and contributes to policy development, including community care planning. The student unit based in the project provides social and community work placements for local courses, and staff contribute to teaching on these courses as well as providing education and training for volunteers and community organizations. The Barton Project moved into purpose built accommodation, alongside a range of statutory and voluntary agencies, and close to the local family centre. These new facilities are the result of years of campaigning by residents and local groups who have been actively involved in planning the centre, a degree of local involvement which has developed over time. In fact, the project's credibility with local people and concerned professionals has been built up over the past two decades.

Although community work has been advocated as an approach to social work since at least 1968, with the Seebohm Report which preceded the establishment of local authority social service departments, the record of implementation has been problematic. As has already been suggested (Hadley *et al.* 1987) progress has been uneven. Furthermore, where community workers have been employed in local authority social service departments, there have been complaints of isolation and marginalization. The study of local authority community work by Davies and Crousaz, for instance, concluded that the majority of community workers had a 'poor relationship with their social work colleagues who appeared to make little effort to learn about community work' (Davies and Crousaz 1982: xvii) and their 'peripheral situation in the organisation and their detachment from the main hierarchy was more disadvantage than benefit to community work in most of the agencies studied' (p. xviii).

Experience so far has been that despite arguments about the logic of developing preventive, community based approaches, in practice the immediate demands of statutory work, such as child protection, take precedence in the allocation of scarce resources. In particular, in some areas, there has been increasing pressure upon the more generalist types of preventive community work (concerned with issues such as the development of anti-poverty strategies). Similarly, despite the logic of increasing support for the voluntary and informal sectors, including community work support, in the current context of community care policies in the mixed economy of welfare, the reality has been the reverse. The National Council for Voluntary Organisations has estimated that over the financial year 1990/91 to 1991/92, the voluntary sector, overall, suffered cuts of £30 million in real terms (NCVO 1992).

Unrealistic expectations have also been identified as a source of problems for community work. Studies of community work in practice have explored gaps between rhetoric and reality (e. g. Barr 1991; Van Reenon 1991:210–19). More fundamentally, in terms of contemporary debates, Abrams and others have argued that there are realistic limits to the potential for developing neighbourhood based, informal community care, and that community work can and does also lead to increased demands for statutory services. Government policies attempting to reduce public provision were, they argued, 'leading to more bureaucratic control of voluntary care, the aim being the provision of officially approved services' (Abrams *et al.* 1989:74). Ultimately, such an approach to partnership between statutory and voluntary sectors and between statutory and community work more generally, risks being self-defeating.

Meanwhile, the problems associated with colonization have not been confined to community work, in relation to community care. There have been wider anxieties that the contracting process, within the mixed economy of welfare, could distort the entire development of the voluntary sector, squeezing out the smaller, more informal community organizations, and reducing the voluntary sector's advocacy role in favour of direct service provision (Gutch 1992). In parallel, there have been anxieties that community work may be increasingly focused upon community based service provision, too, at the expense of community workers' roles as change agents in promoting community participation and empowerment. Community workers face potential conflicts in being accountable to their employers while serving communities who may have divergent agendas. The government's Community Development Project (1969–78) provided examples of these types of conflict in practice. One of the reasons why government support was withdrawn from CDP was that project workers articulated criticisms of government policies to tackle poverty and deprivation and supported community and trade union campaigns for change (Green 1992).

The contemporary context for community work is more contradictory than ever. Current policies towards enabling local authorities, with greater emphasis upon the role of the community sector, within the mixed economy of welfare, would suggest the need for a significant expansion of community work, both within statutory and voluntary agencies. And similarly, greater emphasis upon user participation would seem to indicate an enhanced role for community work, both within social services and within the wider range of welfare service provision. But meanwhile, resources are being squeezed for all but the more pressing statutory areas of work, and there is increasing centralization of decision making, a process which is effectively taking power away from democratically accountable local authorities and from local communities.

Community work can be promoted and has been promoted for widely differing reasons, ranging from strategies to facilitate the substitution of unpaid, informal care for essential public service provisions, through to strategies to combat poverty and oppression, and to promote community empowerment and social transformation. While community work can be developed in such different ways, professional community work's identity and values can perhaps provide some safeguards against abuses; the values of particular relevance here include professional respect for individuals and community groups' rights to self-determination, and professional respect for the principles and practice of equal opportunities.

By itself, community work cannot possibly substitute for wider processes of economic, social and political change, in whichever direction these changes are targeted. But community work does have the potential to contribute to such wider processes of change, and especially so in relation to the development of more preventive and more participatory approaches to social work, within the framework of alternative policies to promote more appropriate, more co-ordinated and more democratically accountable approaches to economic and social planning, to meet social needs.

REFERENCES

Abrams, P., Abrams, S., Humphrey, R. and Snaith, R. (1989) *Neighbourhood Care and Social Policy*, London: HMSO.
Association of Metropolitan Authorities (1989) *Community Development: The Local Authority Role*, London: AMA.
Bamford, T. (1990) *The Future of Social Work*, London: Macmillan.
Barclay Committe (1982) *Social Workers: Their Role and Tasks*, London: National Institute for Social Work/Bedford Square Press.

78   *Practising social work*

Barr, A. (1991) *Practising Community Development*, London: Community Development Foundation.
Batten, T. (1967) *The Non-Directive Approach in Group and Community Work*, Oxford: OUP.
Bulmer, M. (1987) *The Social Basis of Community Care*, London: George Allen and Unwin.
Butcher, H. (1992) 'Community work: current realities, contemporary trends', in P. Carter, T. Jeffs and M. Smith (eds) *Changing Social Work and Welfare*, Buckingham: Open University Press.
Community Work Group (1973) *Current Issues in Community Work*, London: Routledge & Kegan Paul.
Citizen's Charter (1991) London: HMSO.
Clarke, R. (ed.) (1990) *Enterprising Neighbours: The Development of the Community Association Movement in Britain*, London: National Federation of Community Organisations.
Davies, C. and Crousaz, D. (1982) *Local Authority Community Work: Realities of Practice*, London: HMSO.
Filkin, E. and Naish, M. (1982) 'Whose side are we on? The damage done by neutralism', in G. Craig, N. Derricourt and M. Loney (eds) *Community Work and the State*, London: Routledge & Kegan Paul.
Gibbons, J. and Thorpe, S. (1989) *Family Support and Prevention: Report to the Joseph Rowntree Foundation*, London: National Institute for Social Work.
Green, J. (1992) 'The Community Development Project revisited', in P. Carter, T. Jeffs and M. Smith (eds) *Changing Social Work and Welfare*, Buckingham: Open University Press.
Griffiths, Sir Roy (1988) *Community Care: Agenda for Action*, London: HMSO.
Gulbenkian Foundation (1969) *Community Work and Social Change*, Harlow: Longman.
Gutch, R. (1992) *Contracting: Lessons from the US*, London: National Council for Voluntary Organisations.
Hadley, R., Cooper, M., Dale, P. and Stacy, G. (1987) *A Community Social Worker's Handbook*, London: Tavistock.
Harlesden Community Project (1979) *Community Work and Caring for Children: A Community Project in an Inner City Local Authority*, Ilkley: Owen Wells.
Holman, R. (1983) *Resourceful Friends*, London: The Children's Society.
Hope, A. and Timmel, S. (1984) *Community Workers' Handbook*, Gweru, Zimbabwe: Mambo Press.
Loney, M. (1983) *Community against Government*, London: Heinemann Educational Books.
NCVO News, 1992, Jan/Feb, no. 31, London: NCVO.
Seebohm Committee (1968) *Report of the Committee on Local Authority and Allied Social Services*, London: HMSO.
Twelvetrees, A. (1991) *Community Work*, London: Macmillan.
Van Reenon, L. (1991) 'Discrepancies in the working time of community workers', *Community Development Journal* 26(3): 210–19.

FURTHER READING

Adams, R. (1990) *Self Help, Social Work and Empowerment*, London: Macmillan.

Astin, B. (1979) 'Linking an information centre to community development' in M. Dungate (ed.) *Collective Action*, Newcastle upon Tyne: Association of Community Workers.

Baldock, P. (1974) *Community Work and Social Work*, London: Routledge & Kegan Paul.

Broady, M. and Hedley, R. (1989) *Working Partnerships: Community Development in Local Authorities*, London: Bedford Square Press.

Chanan, G. (1991) *Taken For Granted: Community Activity and the Crisis of the Voluntary Sector*, London: Community Development Foundation.

Craig, G., Derricourt, N. and Loney, M. (1982) *Community Work and the State – Towards a Radical Practice*, London: Routledge & Kegan Paul.

Henderson, P. and Thomas, D. (1983) *Skills in Neighbourhood Work*, London: George Allen and Unwin.

Ohri, A., Manning, B. and Curno, P, (eds) (1982) *Community Work and Racism*, London: Routledge & Kegan Paul.

6 The behavioural approach to social work

John Pierson

Social work has long regarded behaviour modification with considerable suspicion as a form of social engineering based on an instrumental view of human nature at odds with the emphasis which the profession places on the whole person, the quality of relationships and client self-determination.

This suspicion is not unfounded. Much of the work on learning theory early in this century which provided the theoretical basis for the behavioural approach seems in retrospect a dangerous abridgement of how people learn behaviours. Early attempts at treatment were cold and detached: a paper from the 1940s entitled 'Operant conditioning of a vegetative human organism' captures the harsh language behaviourists routinely employed (Fuller 1949, cited by Remington 1991). The token economy programmes of the 1950s and 1960s cast psychiatric nurses as behavioural engineers; crude implementation of reward and punishment schemes often had to do more with control over a resident population than individual treatment. Further, the pronounced antagonism from some behaviourists toward homosexuality revealed a rigid attitude toward sexual identity.

But that is not the whole picture. In the last ten years a more pragmatic behavioural approach has begun to emerge, one more sensitive to user choice and partnership. Learning theory has continued to evolve; it now takes account of mind and language as important shapers of behaviour and is more frequently found integrated with systems and interactional theory.

There are four broad characteristics of the behavioural approach. First, behaviour is viewed as functional for the individual, including behaviour which is excessive, challenging or poorly adapted to the social environment. The approach therefore rejects a disease model in which behaviour is seen as a symptom of a deeper disturbance. Second, it concentrates on specific and observable behaviour of the present rather than looking for psychological roots in the past. Third, intervention is aimed at change and must provide opportunities to learn other behaviours. Undesirable behaviours are part of a continuum; they are learned and therefore can be unlearned. Fourth, the approach is held accountable through a strong commitment to evaluating the effectiveness of specific techniques. This accountability introduces a dynamic factor into the behavioural approach which aspires to improved effectiveness.

Learning theory, which underpins the behavioural approach, is a set of assumptions about how people learn behaviour. From the outset in the United States in the early part of this century it employed a language that tried to imitate the natural sciences with words like stimulus, response, conditioning, extinction. Much of this language, developed in relation to laboratory work with animals, is still employed by behaviourists. But while the original terminology has remained it now embraces a wider, more complex range of phenomena and thus is easily misunderstood. Stimulus, for instance, can refer among other things to an event, a sound, words, a sensory experience, verbal rules, another person's behaviour.

The early learning theorists invariably began their work with animals from which they discovered their central premise: a rat's pleasure in finding food, or in escaping from confinement, would teach it to repeat the behaviour that achieved that end. Conversely, it would learn to avoid behaviour that brought about unpleasant consequences.

Learning theorists endeavoured to transfer such insights to the human world. The American J. B. Watson was among the most zealous. He saw all human behaviour entirely in terms of conditioned experiences:

> Give me a dozen healthy infants, well-formed, and my own specified world to bring them up in and I'll guarantee to take any one at random and train him to become any type of specialist I might select – doctor, lawyer, artist... regardless of his talents, penchants, abilities, vocations, and race of his ancestors.
>
> (Watson 1931, cited in Walker 1984)

Watson popularized a version of classical conditioning which the Russian psychologist Pavlov discovered in relation to animals: he succeeded in inducing a phobia of rats in 18-month-old 'little Albert' by repeatedly putting a rat in the boy's playpen and simultaneously banging a four foot long steel bar behind the boy's head with a hammer. This instance of abuse – his planned deconditioning never took place – is still sometimes cited without comment in text books.

His doctrine radically downgraded the importance of both the mind and the emotions in shaping behaviour. Although he was criticized at the time by more flexible, indeed interesting behaviourists such as E. C. Tolman, for 'muscle twitchism', Watson exerted an enormous influence. He wrote a best seller on rearing children, and left his mark on, among others, Bertrand Russell and Aldous Huxley in *Brave New World*. Eventually he left his university post in the 1920s to join a New York advertising firm for $70,000, then a fabulous sum of money (Walker 1984).

The notion of pairing stimuli, however, did in time provide one of the major techniques of behavioural psychotherapy called systematic desensitization whereby the therapist takes a person suffering from anxiety or phobia through a relaxation routine at the same time as imagining or being exposed in actuality to the anxiety provoking source.

B. F. Skinner's influence has been more substantial than any other theorist. From the 1930s to the 1960s his version of behaviourism dominated the field. Skinner was interested in voluntary behaviour. From his many experiments with pigeons he reached the conclusion that most behaviour is developed and modified by its consequences. He called this 'operant' behaviour because it operates on the environment. Consequences that cause behaviours to increase he called 'reinforcers' and those that cause behaviours to decrease 'punishers'. By studying animal behaviour in relation to these twin forces he believed he had discovered a universal law of 'operant conditioning'.

His insight that the consequences of particular behaviours guide a person's future behaviour was profound and pervasive. Several key concepts developed from this thinking. 'Negative reinforcement' refers to a process in which the removal of an unpleasant stimulus (i. e. a thing, activity, other person's behaviour) will increase the probability that the behaviour which brought about that removal will be repeated. Skinner also thought that if a response is reinforced every time it occurs, the behaviour will quickly revert when that reinforcement stops. On the other hand, behaviour inconsistently or 'partially' reinforced is more likely to persist – a principle of which gamblers are all too aware.

By the 1960s, however, psychologists were beginning to acknowledge that learning behaviour was a more complex process than simply through the reinforcing or punishing of specific behaviours. What was obvious to common sense gradually became apparent to learning theorists, although by no means all: the power of the mind in shaping behaviour could no longer be ignored.

The acquisition of language was one area where there was considerable dispute. Behaviourists like Skinner seemed to be saying that language was learned as other physical behaviours through a process of cumulative reinforcement. Anti-behaviourists, such as the linguist Noam Chomsky (1959), pointed out that life was not long enough for the process to happen in this way.

In the 1970s learning theorists split into different orientations and are now fragmented into largely irreconcilable camps. Alongside unreconstructed Skinnerians are cognitive behaviourists such as Meichenbaum (1977) who saw behaviour shaped by thoughts, images, internal verbal statements and self-instructions. Social learning theorists, such as Albert Bandura (1977), emphasized that learning behaviour is a social act, acquired through modelling, imitation and observation.

The history of learning theory, then, is one of coming to terms with its own early rigidities. The nature of reinforcement changed from being a factor which essentially elicits and strengthens a behaviour in an automatic way, to one which serves principally as an informant in deciding a course of action. Self-reinforcement and notions of self-efficacy, achievement and symbolic satisfactions were finally acknowledged as important factors in individual behaviour. Bandura (1977) wrote, 'Humans do not simply respond to stimuli: they interpret them.'

By the 1980s the time of universal psychological theories such as Skinner's, accounting for all behaviour, thought and emotion, was probably over. Psychologists were increasingly looking at the mind as consisting of a large number of independent systems which operate in parallel, with each specifically keyed to a certain kind of information and governing certain kind of behaviours and competences (Gardner 1985). The most convincing work in learning theory now is found in the form of behavioural mini-theories which aim to account for specific sets of problems but do not claim universal status. Gerald Patterson's work, elegantly interweaving social learning, systems and interactional theories (1982, 1988), is one example of a pragmatic but carefully measured attempt to explain the familial conditions in which aggression in young boys is shaped over time.

Despite the limitations of learning theory a behavioural social work practice has developed over the last twenty-five years with a number of distinctive elements to it. A behavioural *assessment* begins with an exploration of problems. It is important to resist the temptation to identify obvious deficits in behaviour of particular individuals as the source of problems. Increasingly the approach recognizes that users, parents or other family members and advocates have the primary interest in defining problems. Assessment is not a question of professional analysis but ultimately one of values, prioritizing those the resolution of which will contribute most to improving a person's quality of life.

Once a problem has been prioritized it is imperative to generate possible solutions, and if particular behaviours are acknowledged by clients, carers or family members as requiring change in order to resolve a designated problem, some element of a behavioural intervention may be indicated. This phase of the assessment is not complete until a target behaviour is specified: what it is, who is doing it, the conditions under which the person is expected to perform that behaviour, and whether it is to be increased or decreased.

It is critical to establish a *baseline* – the rate at which the specific behaviour occurs before intervention. Different methods are used for taking such measurements: self-reports, the observation of those living with or working with the client, or by direct observation by the practitioner. Measuring a behaviour requires defining that behaviour accurately, deciding who will do the observing and ensuring that person has the skills to observe and record accurately. The more minute the selected behaviour, for example eye contact between an autistic child and an adult, the more complex the job of measuring becomes.

Whatever the means the measurement should be quantified. Usually the results are expressed in graph form with the number of occurrences of the target behaviour plotted on the vertical axis and the time span (usually the number of days or hours) of observation plotted along the horizontal axis. Of course measurement continues after a programme has begun; the whole point of establishing a baseline is to measure any subsequent progress in either diminishing or increasing a particular behaviour.

The final element of a behavioural assessment is *functional analysis* which attempts to discover the purpose that a particular behaviour serves for an individual. A person may engage in two behaviours that seem very different – for example, self-injury and aggression – but analysis may show that they serve a similar purpose. The individual employs the problematic behaviour in order to meet certain needs or desires. Although viewed as challenging, self-injurious or anti-social by other persons, the fact that it is used by the individual at a high rate suggests that it is a reasonably effective strategy in that environment. Functional analysis looks to answer the question why or how a behaviour makes sense to the individual and how its purpose may be achieved by an alternative behaviour.

The purpose of functional analysis is to track those factors which shape a particular behaviour. Behaviourists often refer to an 'A–B–C' analysis: noting the *antecedents*, that is the events or circumstances which preceded the behaviour which may act as triggers; the intensity and duration of the *behaviour* itself; and the *consequences* of that behaviour. The standard way of recording this information is through an 'ABC' chart which simply logs the information under each heading in parallel columns. In practice the observer's recording begins when the selected behaviour is observed. Then careful note is made of all consequences of that behaviour with a view to isolating those consequences that act as reinforcers. The last step is to recall what was happening when the person engaged in the selected behaviour, for example the actions of a carer or family member, the setting of a task, the entrance of another person into the room, or a sensory stimulation.

Since behavioural assessment can be rigorous and time consuming, pragmatic judgements have to be made regarding duration, complexity and choice of personnel. Take as an example the assessment of a 4-year-old child who has been referred for behaviour problems. It typically begins with an interview with the parents to establish what behaviours the child is showing and how these are a problem. This is done in as descriptive a way as possible avoiding unclear phrases, such as 'hyperactive' or 'he misbehaves', which are inferential and open to varied, even conflicting interpretation. Some of the possible determinants of the behaviour would be looked at in conjunction with the parents – such as the type and extent of parental involvement with the child and their attitude to giving reward and punishment.

As part of the process of problem definition and establishing a baseline of target behaviours parents would complete a rating scale which quantifies both the intensity of behaviours and the degree of distress these cause. One of the most common is the Eyberg Child Behaviour Inventory (Eyberg and Ross 1978) which asks the parent to record how often the child displays a number of specific problem behaviours, such as refusing to follow a command until threatened with punishment, on a scale from 1 (never) to 7 (always). It also asks which of these behaviours are a problem for the parent.

Some direct observation by the practitioner of the parents playing with the child over a period of between 30 and 60 minutes may also be required. This could involve three components: parents letting the child take the lead in play activity, parents asking the child to play with something else, and parents asking the child to put the toys away. Of particular interest is the parents' use of warning, the kind of commands issued, the use of threats and sanctions for non-compliance and rewards for compliance.

A behavioural assessment of a person with severe learning difficulties would be very different. Greater emphasis may be placed on functional analysis to determine what purpose a particular behaviour has for the individual and whether there are alternative behaviours or skills that could achieve the same end more effectively. Family members, members of staff and others who have frequent contact with the individual may have ideas as to what the specific behaviour achieves and these need to be explored. Some form of trial and error with the setting may be required to discover what the behaviour is actually trying to signal.

For example, after 15 minutes of work at a particular task a man begins yelling and throwing materials on the floor and then runs away. This may be because he has tired of the task and lost self-control, or because the task is too difficult, or because he dislikes someone he is working with. Assessment often highlights a reciprocity between problem behaviours and more effective behaviours; once the function of a behaviour is established a programme which provides an alternative way of achieving the same objective may be built up.

Behavioural *intervention* seeks to modify selected behaviours or to teach new behaviours using techniques based on learning theory.

The simplest way to increase particular behaviours, according to operant procedures, is to reinforce the person engaging in that behaviour. A reinforcer can be something tangible, such as toys, trips, preferred activities, preferred foods, or intangible such as attention, praise, a hug, personal satisfaction, increased effectiveness.

A reinforcer may be particular to the individual and not at all resemble the stereotypical 'reward'. For instance, behaviours performed at a higher rate can be used to reinforce those performed at a lower rate on the assumption that a frequently performed behaviour is sufficiently attractive to the individual to act as a reinforcer. By definition a reinforcer is whatever increases the likelihood that the behaviour which it follows will be performed again. Most behavioural interventions are built on the systematic use of reinforcers to increase desired behaviours and the occasional use of low-level punishers such as time out. In behavioural language this is called 'contingency management'.

If reinforcing desirable behaviours is the cornerstone of behaviour modification it is also the source of the controversy that has raged over the approach since its inception. There is increasing sensitivity within the field that reinforcers should represent typical and natural consequences that are generally available in the individual's environment and that they must be appropriate in terms of age, gender and culture. Understanding what constitutes an appropriate reinforcer, one that is considered worth working for by the individual concerned, requires careful analysis in its own right. Any reinforcement should be made immediately after the selected behaviour, consistently applied and given with conviction.

From this basic operant procedure a number of other techniques follow. The concept of *shaping* means reinforcing approximate attempts at performing a selected behaviour, and subsequently reinforcing those efforts which more closely conform to the final desired behaviour. *Chaining* means reinforcing completion of parts of a more complex behaviour such as a skill, task or activity, until the entire chain of components are linked together in a continuous behaviour. Forward chaining begins with the first component, linking further training to its successful completion. Backward chaining begins with the final component first and works backwards towards the beginning of the sequence. It is generally regarded as more effective because it uses the consequence of completion as a reinforcement in its own right (Tsoi and Yule 1987).

Other techniques flow from social learning theory and are less concerned with manipulating the environment around the individual than teaching specified skills that bring at least partial mastery of that environment. The principal technique is *modelling*: a person who has already mastered a particular skill demonstrates it for another who wishes to learn the same response. The sequence can be as complex or as simple as required.

Modelling combined with chaining is commonly used to master a broad range of self-help and social skills, from basic tasks such as purchasing items in a shop, to handling more complex social situations such as interviews. A successful programme depends on breaking the skill into component parts through *task analysis*, and providing rehearsal and feedback to the person as each component is tried. The objective is a form of stimulus control where the completion of one component acts as a cue to begin the next component.

In practice interventions take on very different constructions. As an example of the slow and painstaking work often involved, Hemsley and Carr (1987) have outlined a programme for a young boy with learning difficulties who is hyperkinetic and unable to sit still for even a few minutes. It is impossible to teach him any constructive activities such as doing puzzles, to sit for meals, or to learn toilet training. His speech is non-existent. The first stage is to set an appropriate behavioural goal, one that is both realistic and which those in daily contact with the boy – primarily teachers and parents – can agree on. They agree on a goal that is modest but attainable: to have the boy sit still for one minute and listen to instructions. Upon this other behaviour can be built. Reinforcers are chosen that are attractive enough to override the boy's continuous motion. The boy is then taught sitting. In a room free of other distractions he is asked to sit down and then held and seated on the chair. Immediately he is praised and given a crisp and a cuddle. The process continues in short sessions of no more than ten minutes with some ten to twenty attempts at the task, each reinforced. After a week it is clear that the boy probably does not understand the meaning of 'sit down' but nevertheless does it in expectation of a reward.

Working with the parents of children who have behavioural problems – such as excessive tantrums, acts of aggression, a high rate of non-compliance with parental commands – requires a different type of intervention, broadly called parent management training, which in essence helps parents to apply the basic principles of learning theory to the management of their own children (Scott 1988; Elliott 1992; Kazdin 1987).

The programmes, though varied, tend to follow a common sequence. The parents are introduced at the beginning to the elements of the behavioural approach itself and in particular the power of negative reinforcement to generate and escalate unwanted behaviours. The so-called 'negative reinforcement trap' clarifies how it is that the parent–child interaction can have very different short-and long-term outcomes; it has, in effect, a double pay-off. For example a parent asks the child to put its toys away. The child refuses and the parent tells the child off in angry tones. The child begins to whine or cry. The parent stops the telling off and the child stops crying. Both have behaved in such a way as to maximize short-term gains – the scolding and the crying stop. Both behaviours have been negatively reinforced in the sense that each was able to terminate unpleasant ('aversive') events. But the room remains untidy and the child has learned how to avoid the task although next time may have to escalate the behaviour.

Subsequent sessions aim to teach specific skills based on learning principles. One of the most important is making commands work. Parental commands are only effective if parents learn how to follow through after issuing them. A taught sequence of steps helps make this happen: compliance should be rewarded immediately (within seconds) with a positive response from the adult, such as praise or approval. If the child has not complied the command should be repeated. Arguing, protesting, whining, crying are all evasive behaviours and should be ignored. Parents also learn not to make too many or difficult commands; after all, on average, all children avoid one command out of three.

Parent training sessions also look at learning to ignore unwanted behaviour and the careful use of 'time out' which, in behavioural terms, means 'time out from positive reinforcement'. This often misunderstood concept should last no more than three to five minutes during which time the child should be placed in a neutral space within view.

Considerable use is made of 'homework': parents apply the techniques and report back at the following session. The training does, therefore, make considerable demands on the participants and a certain percentage do drop out (Elliott 1992). A number of manuals, detailed programmes and at least one extensive set of trigger videotapes for use in a group format provide key tools for participants and practitioners (Webster-Stratton 1991).

In working with adults with severe learning difficulties the objective of intervention may be to reduce or extinguish challenging or 'excess' behaviours, euphemisms denoting anything from socially inappropriate behaviour, such as taking off clothes in public places, to acts of self-injurious behaviour or aggression. A programme is built either around removing identified reinforcements which the unwanted behaviour is obtaining or by reinforcing another behaviour which is incompatible with the unwanted behaviour and in time will replace it. This latter process is known as the differential reinforcement of other behaviour (DRO). For example, a DRO programme to deal with hand biting might involve providing something the person likes, say a pat on the shoulder or a short conversation, for every two minutes in which no biting occurred.

It makes little sense to diminish certain unwanted behaviours without building up social skills. For teaching a specific activity or skill to enhance personal effectiveness in the community the programme is very different – moving from basic to increasingly complex simulations as greater attention is paid to the different types of cues that an individual can expect to encounter. Albin *et al.* (1987) outline four broad steps in developing such a programme:

1 Define the instructional environment in terms of the variations in conditions that the person will encounter.

2 Define the range of relevant stimulus and response variation – when teaching activities in natural settings there is often a range of stimuli or cues that point to appropriate responses; this variation in what to expect as well as the range of appropriate behaviours in response both have to be taught.

3 Select examples for teaching – including those that sample the full range of responses as well as what not to do.

4 Sequence teaching examples – determine the order in which examples are to be taught.

For example, a person undertaking a purchase at a fast food restaurant would encounter a number of stimuli: a door with other people entering or leaving, a counter, assistants taking orders, people waiting in a queue, an assistant asking for the order, the position of the till. Each requires a possible range of response: how to move up in the queue, when to give an order, where to pay and how much. Teaching combines simulation in settings where the cues will approximate those found in the natural setting as closely as possible and natural settings. Staff undertaking such teaching need a variety of skills – task analysis, pacing the instruction in sessions, recognizing the help levels required such as the degree of guidance and prompting, and the capacity to deliver appropriate feedback and reinforcements.

Evaluating the usefulness of the behavioural approach for social work raises a number of points.

First, despite the misplaced enthusiasm of some proponents the approach does not offer a universal social work method. What suits the clinician does not necessarily suit the social worker. The exclusive focus on behaviour makes the approach difficult to adapt to the general run of social work tasks which are dominated by care management, protective functions and the pressure to ration support services. While the specific skills are well within the grasp of social workers the approach does demand considerable time and consistency of purpose and is therefore more adapted to specialist social work settings, including residential environments, where some access to, or collaboration with, a clinical psychologist is available.

Second, for all that the approach acknowledges that behaviour is functional to a given person in a given environment, it sheds no light on how behaviour can be constructed, and distorted, by pressures which arise from structural and cultural forces. An explicitly anti-discriminatory practice is difficult within the behaviouralist perspective alone since ultimately it relies on broad and often unspecified notions of norms for behaviour which are taken uncritically from the dominant culture. A number of writers have underscored how important it is for any social work approach to recognize that individuals who are confronted by a dominant set of cultural norms because of their race, culture, or ethnicity are forced to adapt to two very different, often conflicting, cultures at the same time – their own and that of the dominant culture. What appears to be 'maladaptive' or 'dysfunctional' from a behaviouralist point of view can be the consequence of the struggle to create family systems that can survive the impact of a hostile external environment (Freeman 1990; de Anda 1984).

Third, the behavioural approach has a legacy of professional paternalism which was a result of the techniques spreading rapidly in the 1960s without any concern for the values and attitudes of those who acquired them (Kiernan 1991). Nowhere is this more evident than in work with adults with learning difficulties where the contest between behaviouralists on the one hand, and advocates and groups of users supporting normalization goals on the other, has been extremely heated. There are some signs that behaviouralists are willing to admit to past insensitivities, with some further signs that any intervention should directly augment a person's functioning in the community (Felce 1991).

There are considerable strengths, however, to be placed alongside these limitations. The approach aims to produce observable, measurable results. Moreover, the techniques it uses to achieve these results are clear and easily understood. In the coming contract culture where social work increasingly will be called upon to explain more precisely what it is doing and how it is doing it, these two assets will make the approach more, not less, attractive. The precision in describing problems in terms of antecedents–behaviour–consequences serves as a useful corrective to a professional culture which has for too long relied on inferential and woolly terminology.

The approach does suggest specific responses to specific, carefully assessed problems. There is no reason *per se* why it should remain the preserve of the clinician and not the social worker. Indeed as a street-level professional the social worker may be ideally placed to add the perspectives of partnership and user choice. Working with parents and children with behavioural problems provides a good example of behavioural work at its most effective: a proven format, based on partnership and joined to clear techniques. But if social workers are to take up their place in this, or in any other behavioural work, it requires detailed, specialist knowledge and practitioner and agency commitment of a kind now only infrequently found.

ACKNOWLEDGEMENT

The author is grateful to Dr Jonathan Hill, Professor of Child and Adolescent

Psychiatry, University of Liverpool, and Linda Butler, Wrexham Child and Family Service, for assistance in the preparation of this chapter.

REFERENCES

Albin, R., McDonnell, J. and Wilcox, B. (1987) 'Designing interventions to meet activity goals' in B. Wilcox and B. G. Thomas *A Comprehensive Guide to the Activities Catalog*, Baltimore: Paul Brookes Publishing.

Bandura, A. (1977) *Social Learning Theory*, Englewood Cliffs, New Jersey: Prentice Hall.

Chomsky, N. (1959) Review of Skinner's *Verbal Behaviour, Language* 35: 26–58.

deAnda, D. (1984) 'Bicultural socialisation: factors affecting the minority experience', *Social Work* 29: 101–07.

Elliot, C. (1992) Intervention with young conduct-disordered children: an evaluation of parents' groups, unpublished paper.

Eyberg, S. M. and Ross, A. W. (1978) 'Assessment of child behaviour problems: the validation of a new inventory', *Journal of Clinical Child Psychology* 7: 113–16.

Felce, D. (1991) 'Using behavioural principles in the development of effective housing services for adults with severe or profound mental handicap', in B. Remington (ed.) *The Challenge of Severe Mental Handicap: A Behaviour Analytic Approach*, Chichester: John Wiley and Sons.

Freeman, E. (1990) 'The Black family's life cycle: operationalising a strengths perspective', in S. M. L. Logan, E. M. Freeman and R. G. McRoy (1990) *Social Work Practice With Black Families: A Culturally Specific Perspective*, New York: Longman.

Fuller, R. J. (1949) 'Operant conditioning of a vegetative human organism', *American Journal of Psychology* 62: 587–90.

Gardner, H. (1985) *Frames of Mind: The Theory of Multiple Intelligences*, New York: Basic Books.

Hemsley, R. and Carr, J. (1987) 'Ways of increasing behaviour: reinforcement' in W. Yule and J. Carr (eds) *Behaviour Modification for People with Mental Handicaps*, 2nd edn, London: Chapman & Hall.

Kazdin, A. (1987) 'Treatment of antisocial behaviour in children: current status and future directions', *Psychological Bulletin* 102: 187–203.

Kiernan, C. (1991) 'Professional ethics: behaviour analysis and normalisation' in B. Remington (ed.) *The Challenge of Severe Mental Handicap: A Behaviour Analytic Approach*, Chichester: John Wiley and Sons.

Meichenbaum, D. (1977) *Cognitive-Behaviour Modification: An Integrative Approach*, New York: Plenum Press.

Patterson, G. (1982) *Coercive Family Process*, Eugene, Oregon: Castalia Publishing.

Patterson, G. (1992) *Antisocial Boys*, Eugene, Oregon: Castalia Publishing.

Remington, B. (1991) 'Research and application', in B. Remington (ed.) *The Challenge of Severe Mental Handicap: A Behaviour Analytic Approach*, Chichester: John Wiley and Sons.

Scott, M. (1988) *A Cognitive-Behavioural Approach to Clients' Problems*, London: Tavistock.

Tsoi, M. and Yule, W. (1987) 'Building up new behaviours: shaping, prompting and fading' in W. Yule and J. Carr (eds) *Behaviour Modification for People with Mental Handicaps*, 2nd edn, London: Chapman and Hall.

Walker, Stephen (1984) *Learning Theory and Behaviour Modification*, London: Methuen.
Watson, J. B. (1931) *Behaviourism*, 2nd edn, London: Kegan Paul, Trench and Trubner.
Webster-Stratton, C. (1991) 'Strategies for helping families with conduct disordered children', *Journal of Child Psychology and Psychiatry* 32: 1047–62.

FURTHER READING

Baker, B. *et al.* (1976) *Behaviour Problems*, Champaign, Illinois: Research Press.
Barrowclough, Christine and Fleming, Ian (1990) *Goal Planning with Elderly People*, Manchester: Manchester University Press.
Farrell, Peter, McBrien, Judith, and Foxen, Tom (1992) *Teaching People with Severe Learning Difficulties*, 2nd edn, Manchester: Manchester University Press.
Gibb, Charles and Randall, Peter (1989) *Professionals and Parents: Managing Children's Behaviour*, London: Macmillan Education Ltd.
Hudson, Barbara and Macdonald, Geraldine (1980) *Behavioural Social Work – An Introduction*, London: Macmillan.
McAuley, Roger and McAuley, Patricia (1979) *Child Behaviour Problems – An Empirical Approach to Management*, London: Macmillan.
Meyer, Luanna and Evans, Ian (1989) *Nonaversive Intervention for Behaviour Problems: A Manual for Home and Community*, Baltimore: Paul H. Brookes Publishing Co.
Sheldon, Brian (1982) *Behaviour Modification: Theory, Practice and Philosophy*, London: Tavistock.
Walker, Stephen (1984) *Learning Theory and Behaviour Modification*, London: Methuen.

7 Practising feminist approaches

Annie Hudson with Lorraine Ayensu, Catherine Oadley and Matilde Patocchi

'Feminism' signals to some people very negative images about those who choose to so define themselves; in contrast to others it connotes positive values about women working together to challenge oppressive aspects of their lives. Consequently, it is probably important to emphasize at the outset that this chapter seeks to provide neither an instructional guide to feminist social work practice, nor a series of banner slogans under which the 'converted' may align themselves. We share Hanmer and Statham's view that all too often definitions of feminists and feminism have become exclusive rather than inclusive (Hanmer and Statham 1988) and hope that this discussion will have a purchase on the working day realities of a diverse range of social work practitioners and managers. It is our intention to indicate not only some of the possibilities but also some of the inevitable tensions that result from attempting to translate some of the experiential wisdom accumulated by women collectively into everyday social work practice.

The discussion below draws on our experiences of working together in a social work team in an inner-city area of Bristol. Our relatively diverse social identities and biographies have engendered as much difference as consensus in our ideas about feminist and anti-sexist social work practice. We believe that this is not only a potential strength as opposed to a weakness, but also that it is a reflection of a much broader diversity about the most appropriate means of infusing social work's dominant institutions with the potentially radical concepts implicit within different strands of feminist thought and practice (see, for example, the collection of writings in Langan and Day 1992). Our shared starting point is that feminist analysis can be invaluable for etching out how social workers, including those working in statutory agencies, can begin to address, rather than ignore, the unequal position of women that characterizes so many facets of social relations. Challenging myriad manifestations of gender inequalities, like challenging race, class and other forms of oppression, is, however, an exceedingly complex task. To suggest otherwise would be naive and misleading.

Social workers are confronted daily by the consequences of women's oppression. These may be in the form of witnessing the brutal results of male physical or sexual violence or the more subtle, but equally invidious, manifestations of gender inequalities such as the unquestioned duties felt by many women to care for and about their children, relatives and male partners despite the considerable cost they may accrue for themselves (Dalley 1988). Whilst these are not necessarily new revelations, during the past decade or so feminism has provided social workers with greater clarity and purpose about the imperative of finding ways of challenging and doing something about such inequities, whilst accepting that such endeavours are likely to be relatively piecemeal (see, for example, Marchant and Wearing 1986; Hanmer and Statham 1988; Dominelli and McLeod 1989).

A review of the impact of feminism on social work is particularly timely as the effects of the Children Act 1989 and the National Health Service and Community Care Act 1990 take root in social work agencies. Both Acts contain within them both progressive and regressive potentials as far as the social relations of gender are concerned. Community care policies, with their emphasis on needs-led assessments, on consumer choice and on the duty to consult carers seem superficially to acknowledge the rights and needs of informal carers, the overwhelming majority of whom are women, and also to challenge attitudes that professionals 'know best'. Yet, as many social workers and managers have come to recognize, the 'pluriform care market' ideology (Lupton 1992) that central government has impelled local authorities to stimulate works, in many respects, directly against the needs and interests of women as front-line carers both paid and unpaid. The diversification of relatively cheap community care schemes relies on maintaining women as low paid and low status workers. This trend is likely to intensify as private sector service providers increase their share of the community care 'market', since indications are that private agencies offer less favourable pay and conditions than local government workers have come to receive. Central government statements indicating that aggregated information about unmet needs are unlikely to be officially published has exacerbated concerns that the real needs of community care users and their informal carers will not be credited. The gendered segregation of social services departments means, moreover, that it is largely female staff who are the bearers of messages to users and carers that resources will not meet their needs.

The Children Act 1989 was similarly predicated on traditional views of family life. Whilst also apparently aiming to redress imbalances in professional and state power, the Act barely begins to question structural and institutionalized sources of inequality either within individual families or between families from different social groups (see, for example MacDonald 1991; Langan 1992). It should be noted that the Act makes no reference to the importance of taking account of a child's gender in decision making.

Moreover, the Children Act's underpinning principle of parental partnership implies that parenthood is a genderless concept and reality. Whilst this might be a long-term social policy objective, the reality is that gender defines and shapes virtually every aspect of familial relationships.

The way in which the differential needs and social responsibilities of mothers and fathers respectively are generally subsumed under the sole category of 'parents' is explained in part by the indebtedness of large sections of the Children Act to the *Report of the Inquiry into Child Abuse in Cleveland* (Butler-Sloss 1988). The report failed to highlight either the maleness of most perpetrators or the specific conflicts and dilemmas faced by many women whose children had disclosed sexual abuse by their male partners. Such official silencing of gender in what was arguably one of the key social policy debates of the 1980s is a further illustration of the state's continued denial of the significance of gender, and of the role which white middle-class men so often occupy in gatekeeping and commanding the operations of the welfare 'industry' (Campbell 1988; Hudson 1992).

DEFINING OUR TERMS: WHAT CONSTITUTES FEMINIST APPROACHES?

Feminism has never been an easy concept to identify or to define. Broadly speaking, however, feminism can be regarded as referring to beliefs that all dimensions of social relations are shaped by the structure of power relations between women and men. As such then, feminism provides a template for making sense of the diverse and often contrasting ways in which women experience inequality in so many facets of their lives – at home, at work and in the wider community. Power relations, however, are not simply an issue of some having 'it' and others being without 'it'. Such a view is far too simplistic. What is required instead is careful scrutiny of the specific power relations which may be obtaining in any particular situation and how these impact on the particular women and men involved.

The importance of avoiding simplistic presumptions about the sources and manifestations of gender oppression is highlighted by the very great material and social differences which exist between different groups of women (Lorde 1984; Segal 1987). Feminism has rightly sometimes been castigated for being synonymous with the values and experiences of white, heterosexual and middle-class women. Such a criticism is as valid of many commentaries about social work as elsewhere. That dominant models of feminism have so often been treated with suspicion and anger by many black and working-class women should come as no surprise to anyone (see, for example, Shah 1989).

A number of features have characterized the integration of feminist approaches into social work policy and practice. First, it is evident that feminist approaches are intrinsically threatening to many of social work's traditionally held beliefs. The notion of professional objectivity or neutrality, for example, is disputed by the feminist emphasis on the invariable influence of our values and how they inescapably permeate all that we do both professionally and personally. Mary Eaton's research illustrates such patterns. This indicated that probation officers are likely to use home visits with their female clients to comment and adjudicate upon their domestic competence. In contrast, home visits to male clients were frequently used as an opportunity to learn more about the defendant's domestic relationships rather than his domestic competence. Such findings exemplify how social workers frequently continue to presume the centrality of the domestic role in women's lives and to expect that they should account for their menfolk's actions (Eaton 1986). The impact of such presumptions on child protection policy and practice is discussed later.

Second, endeavours to integrate feminist perspectives into social work have increasingly sought to recognize both the strength and the meaning of diversities between women, as well as the complex nature of power differentials between worker and client. Social work may have begun to address the significance of different forms of oppression but there remains a strong inclination to reduce the complexities of the lives of users to neat little boxes labelled 'race', 'gender', 'class' and so on. The reality of individuals' lives is of course very different. None of us belongs to one social compartment; we are simultaneously female or male, black or white, working class or middle class. That said, each of us has our own very individual biography and understanding of the meaning of all the social categories to which we may belong.

Ahmed's discussion of the shortcomings of feminist accounts about young Asian women is pertinent here. She demonstrates how social workers often simplistically reduce conflicts experienced by some young Asian women to explanations of their preference for white British values over those of their parents (Ahmed 1986). When working with black young women, social workers must therefore ensure that their assessments and intervention revolve around a critical appreciation of the specific impact of racism and class as well as sexism and the young woman's particular relationship with her family.

Similarly, women with disabilities have drawn attention to the exclusion by much mainstream feminism of the experiences of disabled women. Jenny Morris, for example has criticized the tendency (possibly even replicated within parts of this chapter) to consider questions about community care via a focus on women as carers, rather than through an equally important focus on the needs and rights of women who are themselves disabled (Morris 1991). Hughes and Mtezuka make similar points about the needs of older women and emphasize the importance of social work assessments encompassing an appreciation of the strengths and resources which older women have gained from their life experiences (Hughes and Mtezuka 1992).

It is often difficult and possibly even embarrassing to acknowledge the frequency with which many of us (but particularly those of us who are white, middle class and heterosexual) presume that our experiences and values are of universal validity. At times we may have even been driven by a secular version of the moral fervour that propelled many of social work's Victorian foremothers, such as Octavia Hill, into philanthropic action. The danger of such evangelical zeal is no less when it stems from feminist philosophy than when it was Victorian Christian philanthropy. In the 1980s one of the authors began undertaking some research into work with 'troublesome young women'. An initial premise for the research was the importance of affirming young women's rights to determine their own sexuality. With hindsight, however, it is apparent that the dominant model of sexuality underpinning that research analysis was not only heterosexist but also class defined. It was accepted, for example, that adequate, free and accessible contraception resources were a crucial component of maximizing young women's choices, particularly in relation to the possibility of 'premature' motherhood. One consequence of talking more extensively to young women was the acknowledgment that the research premises represented only one version of reality. Early motherhood constitutes, for many working-class young women, a valid and not necessarily negative way of achieving a mature adult status and responsibility. Early motherhood is, in short, a source of joy and pleasure for some young women, contrary to many popular and professional preconceptions (Sharpe 1987).

A further feature of feminist approaches to social work has been an emphasis on the need to develop practice theories and methods which are dynamic and responsive to new insights about power relations. Nowhere has this been more apparent than in child sexual abuse. The recognition that women do, albeit infrequently, sexually abuse children was contrary to what many of us had wanted to believe in the early 1980s. This was profoundly disturbing. The recognition that women could be perpetrators of sexual abuse entailed not only listening to the distress and sense of betrayal by those who had been abused by adult women, but it also meant that we had to face up to the limitations of earlier theorizations of child sexual abuse that developed out of campaigns in the early 1980s against the injustice of sexual abuse. The need to rework earlier feminist conceptualizations about sexual abuse has also necessitated a re-examination of practice methods. It is clear, for example, that social workers must be alert to the possibility of sexual abuse of any child by male and female adults. Similarly, it is also fundamental that intervention with female perpetrators, as with male perpetrators, is based on the need to confront the behaviour and not on individual pathology models since this would be to reproduce the very criticisms which feminists have levelled at traditional perspectives (Hudson 1992).

Finally, feminist approaches have sought to build up a reservoir of practical experience about different ways of responding to the gendered needs of clients and workers more equitably. There is now a substantive body of knowledge and direct experience around a number of different practice areas (see Langan and Day 1992 for a collection of articles around different user, organizational and service delivery issues). In some respects the number of publications available about feminist and anti-sexist practice within Great Britain is a poor reflection of the diversity and extensiveness of endeavours by many women (and some men) to challenge and address gender inequalities in their employing agencies. This may reflect the continued difficulty which feminist ideas have in gaining anything more than passing reference in many quarters of social work (but particularly in senior management and academia).

There have been, and no doubt will continue to be, debates about the relative merits of work with men having a key place on the feminist agenda (Segal 1990). There is a risk that, in expending energies on developing anti-sexist practice with men, women's perspectives, needs and values will once more be occluded from public view and debate. That said, the reality is that men do play very significant emotional and social roles in the lives of many women. To cast them to the shadows of our assessment and intervention is unlikely to assist women. If feminist approaches in social work are to meet with any success, then an exclusive concentration on work with women is ultimately likely to engender only half-hearted solutions. This is an area in which male practitioners, managers and educators have a potentially vital role. They have an unequivocal responsibility to challenge both their own attitudes and practices as well as those of male colleagues and thereby to develop gradually a greater repertoire of wisdom about working with male service users.

The remainder of this chapter examines two specific issues which bring into sharp relief some of the tensions and possibilities of feminist approaches to social work. The tension between control and empowerment objectives is considered, followed by discussion of some of the initiatives which will be needed if women employees in social work organizations are to receive a fairer deal.

EMPOWERMENT OR CONTROL?

Feminism's objective of addressing the many-faceted sources and forms of women's oppression would appear to be at odds with social work's historical origins and with its contemporary role in regulating deviant and dissident individuals and families. Social work's control roles have a number of particular resonances for feminist approaches. First, women's status as gatekeepers of family affairs assigns them the unremitting responsibility of maintaining and supporting the family both at an institutional and individual level. When the state identifies a 'problem' within a particular family, it invariably initially focuses its gaze on women in their roles as primary carers and agents of discipline.

Women are generally presumed to be more culpable than their male partners when their families experience difficulties. Attention is thereby diverted away not only from the impact of male roles but also from structural inequalities emanating from poverty and racism. Child care work evidences such patterns most starkly (Parton 1990). Agency case records and the discourse of child protection case conferences are frequently the mechanisms by which welfare professionals express their views about the culpability of individual women to stimulate, develop and care for their children. Rather than addressing the impact of poverty and the inadequacy of material resources to support women in looking after children it is individual women who are frequently castigated and deemed to have failed.

Social work intervention, in common with the practice of allied welfare institutions such as health and social security, often revolves around the perpetuation of negative associations between the (perceived) sexual behaviour of women clients and their capacity to be 'good mothers'. The 'known fact' that a woman works as a prostitute, for example, is sometimes deployed as an index of her potential to be an incompetent parent even though there is no proven correlation. Similarly, a key determinant in decision making about young women perceived to be 'troublesome' by their families, social workers and other professionals is the extent to which such young women are thought to be, or are 'at risk' of sexual activity and possibly 'promiscuity' (Hudson 1989).

Black women clients are particularly susceptible to negative stereotypes about their capacities to be 'good enough' mothers. Such stereotypes emanate from suppositions about their sexual behaviour. One particularly common-place presumption is that Afro-Caribbean women will frequently have many sexual partners which in turn generates presumptions of their amorality and incompetence to manage the demands of motherhood. Risk assessment checklists used by child protection agencies are frequently simplistic and uncritical, often classifying black families as being 'high risk' particularly when parents are young and single (Channer and Parton 1990). Such images contradict evidence that young Afro-Caribbean mothers tend to have a mature sense of responsibility and ability to cope as mothers (Channer and Parton 1990). Such evidence complements our own experiences of the capacities of the young black women with whom we work, some of whom have themselves been in care. Such young black women may develop important social networks which serve to provide not only social and emotional support and enjoyment, but also positive resistance against myriad difficulties that they may face, whether this is from intrusive welfare officials (including social workers such as ourselves), from male partners or from demanding small children.

In a similar vein, racist stereotypes which portray Asian women as passive and dependent can result in negative constructions about their parenting capacities. An Asian woman who is reluctant to allow her child to play on the street outside, or on the local playground, may find herself at the receiving end of negative judgements by social workers or health visitors who perceive her as inhibiting her children's social development. The reality may of course be very different since the woman may be concerned to protect her children from the endemic racism of many neighbourhoods.

Feminists, in common with other 'radical' social workers, have drawn attention to the way in which the focus on individual 'cases' detracts time and time again from the inadequacy of resources to support women in their private and public roles. In recent years, social work resources have been increasingly prioritized for families defined as 'high risk', thereby confirming the apparently unrelenting shift back to a residual rather than a universalistic model of welfare. It is working-class and minority ethnic families who are the main victims of such 'residualization of local authority services' and who benefit least from the expanding private and voluntary services which cost more than many women can afford (Langan 1992:83).

Black women have particularly limited welfare service choices. The much publicized cases of Asian women being unjustly imprisoned following conviction for killing their violent husbands have highlighted Asian women's extremely limited access to resources which would open up rather than foreclose their options for leaving violent men. In many areas of the country, for example, Asian women have to travel hundreds of miles before they will find a women's refuge that will meet their needs.

Similarly, shortfalls in interpreter services in many social work agencies may particularly penalize Asian women. A significant proportion of Asian women who wish to access welfare services are often reliant on male partners or relatives to communicate with white officials such as social workers, thereby limiting the possibility of their receiving services in their own right and on their own terms.

Empowerment is a concept which has been a *sine qua non* of feminist perspectives, as in other strands of radical social work thinking (Ward and Mullender 1991). Empowerment is none the less a notion about which it is very much easier to theorize and sloganize than to translate into everyday working principles and practice. In statutory agencies particularly, the pressure to 'cover your backs' can easily stifle initiative and risk taking. As already indicated, consumer participation and partnership are ostensibly at the heart of both the Children Act 1989 and the National Health Service and Community Care Act 1990. Yet both pieces of legislation have unequivocally failed to address structural sources of inequality and oppression.

Central to the concept of empowerment in social work is the idea that individuals are not passive victims of their situations. Many facets of the women's movement, such as Women's Aid and Rape Crisis Centres, have demonstrated the effectiveness and power of women developing practical strategies to challenge and alter their circumstances. In social work agencies, empowerment necessarily entails moving away from presumptions that we are 'experts' and that clients should be the passive recipients of our services. A number of projects working with young women 'in trouble' have drawn attention to the potential of encouraging young women to engage in activities which etch out different and non-traditional concepts of youthful femininity (Mountain 1988). Ward and Mullender have similarly argued that self-directed groupwork based on anti-oppressive values can help reject the 'splintering of the public and private' (Ward and Mullender 1991:29).

The successful expansion of the power of women service users is conditional on assessments linking individuals' needs, resources and problems with broader structural dynamics. It is, however, equally crucial that the capacities of adult women are not strengthened at the expense of the safety and security of potentially more vulnerable individuals, such as children, young people or adults with learning disabilities. A key challenge is how best to ensure that women's rights and power are maximized at the same time as challenging other forms of oppression and disadvantage. The undoubted tension between social work's policing roles and the empowerment of women is unlikely to evaporate. Indeed the tension has arguably become intensified in recent years as right-wing welfare ideologies have increased their grip on the financing and operations of social work agencies.

TOWARDS GREATER GENDER EQUITY IN SOCIAL WORK ORGANIZATIONS

At first sight women employees in social work organizations appear to have a relatively strong profile. Women are undoubtedly strongly physically represented within social work organizations, for example 86 per cent of the workforce in English and Welsh social services departments are female (Social Services Inspectorate 1992a). Additionally, at least when compared to some parts of the private sector, female social services staff generally enjoy relatively fair work conditions as far as issues such as fair selection interviewing, maternity leave and the availability of part-time and career break schemes are concerned. At closer sight, however, it becomes clear that the reality is very different. Indeed, as Jane King has pointed out, social services are run mostly by men while surviving and thriving on the goodwill and resilience of legions of women (King 1992). Men have undoubtedly been extremely successful in achieving and consolidating their power, prestige and high pay within social work agencies. In 1990, for example, 88 per cent of directors of social services in England and Wales, and 80 per cent of assistant or divisional directors were male (Social Services Inspectorate 1992a). It is particularly telling that, despite the impact of feminism and equal opportunities policies, there are now virtually no more female directors of social services in England and Wales than were appointed in the early 1970s when those departments were created. Women's employment patterns and relationship to the labour market, historical legacies and presumptions that tend to define 'good managers' in male-orientated terms and differential career values and aspirations are but some of the factors explaining the relative lack of power of female social services staff. Specific groups of women, such as black women and women with disabilities, experience particularly unequal opportunities for organizational power and status. More substantive evidence of and discussion about such patterns can be found elsewhere (see, for example, Howe 1986; Lupton 1992; Social Services Inspectorate 1992a; Social Services Inspectorate 1992b).

Three types of initiative stand out as urgent priorities. First, whilst policy statements are only ever the first step towards organizational equality and justice, many social services departments and voluntary agencies around the country could start with refining much further the bland statements of intent which so often characterize all aspects of their equal opportunities policies. In drawing up concrete and specific action plans, attention must be given to the differential needs of specific social groups of women. Black women managers, for example, have articulated how they are frequently marginalized and by-passed in agencies where power continues to be concentrated in white groups (Social Services Inspectorate 1992a). Domiciliary care staff, such as home care workers, have often had to deal with working in isolation yet also having a high measure of responsibility for which they receive low pay and minimal training or promotional opportunities. These are but two examples of how different groups of women staff will have different needs and priorities, all of which warrant detailed attention by gender and women's equality policies. Sexual harassment policies and procedures must be effectively implemented alongside equality policies if women employees are to feel safe and secure in taking up issues and grievances when they have cause to do so.

Second, the structure and design of jobs within social services departments requires overhauling. Many women staff need more extensive opportunities to enable them to take time off for caring responsibilities at the same time as keeping abreast, through training and other career development activities, of organizational and practice changes. Similarly, it continues to be difficult for many women to work full time alongside managing the demands of their families. More flexible working arrangements and more positive attitudes towards part-time and job-sharing work are strongly indicated. To our knowledge there have not yet been any examples of job-sharing social services directors; the day that event occurs may begin to presage social work organizations that are making full and equitable use of their female staff resources.

Finally, some redefinition of what constitutes a 'good manager' is demanded. Attention has been drawn elsewhere to the subtle and not so subtle ways in which the contributions and resources of female managers are frequently undermined or ignored (see, for example, Walby 1987; Morris 1988). No wonder then that for many women social workers, management does not have the allure that it may do for their male colleagues. The position of female managers is unlikely to be promoted, moreover, by the evolution of what has been termed the 'new managerialist approach' (Lupton 1992) with its emphasis on quantitive performance measures and an explicitly masculinized culture (as manifest, for example, on the need to be 'tough' and commanding in relation to subordinate staff). Recent Social Services Inspectorate reports and initiatives indicate that there is now greater recognition of the need for all agencies to establish and evaluate a range of training and development schemes for potential and actual women managers. The ability and will of agencies to deliver such schemes will, however, be severely tested in the face of other competing priorities such as community care.

Feminist approaches will have to continue to adjust and adapt in response to the changing shape of social work. As already indicated this is not likely to be an easy task given continued assaults on the resourcing of social services agencies. This chapter has sketched out some of the key components of feminist social work practice. This is, however, a very much easier task than realizing feminist principles in everyday social work practice. The demands of doing the 'job' of social work, particularly in large statutory departments, mean that the potential of many of the best of feminist intentions are often quickly blunted. It is consequently extremely important that, as well as constantly scrutinizing our own practice, apparently small steps towards the successful challenge of oppressive values and practices are also recognized and validated.

REFERENCES

Ahmed, S. (1986) 'Cultural racism in work with Asian women and girls', in S. Ahmed, J. Cheetham, and J. Small *Social Work with Black Children and their Families*, London: Batsford.

Butler-Sloss Committee (1988) *Report of the Inquiry into Child Abuse in Cleveland*, London: HMSO.

Campbell, B. (1988) *Unofficial Secrets, Child Sexual Abuse – The Cleveland Case*, London: Virago.

Channer, Y. and Parton, N. (1990) 'Racism, cultural relativism and child protection', in Violence Against Children Study Group, *Taking Child Abuse Seriously*, London: Unwin Hyman.

Dalley, G. (1988) *Ideologies of Caring*, London: Macmillan.

Dominelli, L. and McLeod, E. (1989) *Feminist Social Work*, London: Macmillan.

Eaton, M. (1986) *Justice for Women?*, Milton Keynes: Open University Press.

Hanmer, J. and Statham, D. (1988) *Women and Social Work*, London: Macmillan.

Howe, D. (1986) 'The segregation of women and their work in the personal social services', *Critical Social Policy* 15, Spring, 21–35.

Hudson, A. (1989) '"Troublesome Girls": towards alternative definitions and policies', in M. Cain (ed.) *Growing Up Good*, London: Sage.

Hudson, A. (1992) 'The child sexual abuse "industry"', in M. Langan and L. Day (eds) *Women, Oppression and Social Work*, London: Routledge.

Hughes, B. and Mtezuka, M. (1992) 'Social work and older women', in M. Langan and L. Day (eds) *Women, Oppression and Social Work*, London: Routledge.

King, J. (1992) 'Women: a demographic time bomb', *Community Care*, 2 July, 16–17.

Langan, M. (1992) 'Who cares? Women in the mixed economy of care', in M. Langan and L. Day (eds) *Women, Oppression and Social Work*, London: Routledge.

Langan, M. and Day, L. (eds) (1992) *Women, Oppression and Social Work*, London: Routledge.

Lorde, A. (1984) *Sister Outsider*, Freedom, CA: The Crossing Press.

Lupton, C. (1992) 'Feminism, managerialism, and performance measurement', in M. Langan and L. Day (eds) *Women, Oppression and Social Work*, London: Routledge.

MacDonald, S. (1991) *All Equal Under the Act?* London: National Institute of Social Work.

Marchant, H. and Wearing, B. (eds) (1986) *Gender Reclaimed*, Sydney: Hale and Iremonger.

Morris, B. (1988) 'Tough talking', *Insight*, 27 May, 17–19.

Morris, J. (1991) *Pride Against Prejudice: Transforming Attitudes to Disability*, London: Women's Press.

Mountain, A. (1988) *Womanpower: a Handbook for Women Working with Young Women in Trouble*, Leicester: National Youth Bureau.

Parton, C. (1990) 'Women, gender oppression and child abuse', in Violence Against Children Study Group, *Taking Child Abuse Seriously*, London: Unwin Hyman.

Segal, L. (1987) *Is the Future Female?*, London: Virago.

Segal, L. (1990) *Slow Motion: Changing Masculinities, Changing Men*, London: Virago.

Shah, N. (1989) 'It's up to you sisters: black women and radical social work', in M. Langan and P. Lee (eds) *Radical Social Work Today*, London: Unwin Hyman.

Sharpe, S. (1987) *Falling for Love: Teenage Mothers Talk*, London: Virago Upstarts.

Social Services Inspectorate (1992a) *Women in Social Services: A Neglected Resource*, London: HMSO.
Social Services Inspectorate (1992b) *Promoting Women*, London: HMSO.
Walby, C. (1987) 'Why are so few women working in senior positions?', *Social Work Today*, 16 February, 10–11.
Ward, D. and Mullender, A. (1991) 'Empowerment and oppression: an indissoluble pairing for contemporary social work', *Critical Social Policy* 32, Autumn, 21–30.

8 Alternatives to custody

Norman Tutt

One of the major dilemmas facing the development of new social work practice is that any new approach cannot readily demonstrate its effectiveness by the methods normally available to clinical practice. In clinical practice, even allowing for the ethical problems involved, it is routine to establish trials with matched samples and random allocations. However, social work is much more methodologically complex since by definition it is attempting to respond to users, within their environment and the interaction between the user and their environment. This means that the number of variables involved are beyond management in any 'experimental' situation. This is never more true than in the field of work with offenders, since in this work the 'user' is rarely if ever defined by the social work agency but can be defined by the public, the police, crown prosecutor, and courts and can change dramatically in their status by a decision being reversed by any one of these agencies.

I was taught this lesson early in my career when working in what was then a remand home. Young people whom I assessed in the belief they were delinquent and I had to discover why, would appear in court, where the police might present no evidence or the court find the young person not guilty and the case be dismissed and the young person immediately be redefined as 'normal'. The recent miscarriages of justice within the criminal justice system have highlighted the dramatic reversals which can occur anywhere in the system. The first question which needs to be asked in this chapter is whether alternatives to custody is an approach, formulated and articulated, or merely an aspiration. Alternatively if it is an approach, is it social work?

In 1978 a number of writers joined with me in producing a book, *Alternative Strategies for Coping with Crime* (Tutt 1978). The introduction stated that alternative strategies engulf a number of approaches:

1 Decriminalization – acceptance of 'criminal' behaviour as normal and recognition of legal action as inappropriate.
2 Non-intervention – acceptance of the need for prescribed and limited statutory intervention.

3 Legitimization – developments in practice aimed at strengthening 'informal' practice.

4 Radical intervention – attempts to avoid the traditional institutional response which is seen as damaging.

Since that time progress towards reducing the use of custody for young offenders has been dramatic, as can be seen in Table 8.1.

Table 8.1 Levels of custodial sentences and care orders on juvenile offenders, 1969 to 1991

	Custody	Care	Total
1965	1,336	6,162	7,498
1969	2,646	5,920	8,556
1970	3,102	6,700	9,802
1971	3,209	6,747	9,956
1972	3,810	6,318	10,128
1973	4,396	6,743	11,139
1974	5,277	7,398	12,675
1975	5,933	7,115	13,048
1976	6,754	6,057	12,811
1977	6,876	5,613	12,489
1978[a]	7,378	5,345	12,723
1979[a]	6,967	4,359	11,326
1980	7,700	4,100	11,800
1981	7,900	3,450	11,350
1982	7,400	3,050	10,450
1983	7,900	2,000	8,900
1984	6,900	1,650	8,550
1985	6,200	1,340	7,540
1986	6,500	1,030	5,530
1987	4,100	820	4,920
1988	3,400	460	3,860
1989	2,400	310	2,710
1990	1,700	205	1,905
1991[b]	1,887	–	1,887

Source: Richardson (1990)
[a] It is possible that figures for 1978 are high and those for 1979 low due to delays following offences re-classification
[b] Provisional figure

1980 and 1981 appear to have been the peak of the custodial actions; since then substantial erosion has occurred. However, these figures obscure a number of disturbing features, for example virtually all of these figures relate to young men. Until the introduction of the Criminal Justice Act 1991, young women were protected from custodial sentences. However this may have had the unintended consequence of classifying a number of delinquent young women as mentally ill rather than criminal and led to longer periods of incarceration in psychiatric facilities than equivalent sentences for males. Moreover crude figures on race suggest that black Afro-Caribbean youths are disproportionately represented in custody compared with their white or Asian peers. A recent report from the Home Office (1992) showed that race is a significant feature in determining if a young man is to be held in custody on remand or receive a custodial sentence.

Over the past decade, social work methods have become refined and the process can now be described in some detail and therefore generalized. The ability to generalize to new (geographical) areas or different user groups is the hallmark whereby activity can be defined as a method. There are four key elements to the process:

1 The development of local policies with clear objectives, strategies and targets, preferably agreed with the other agencies which constitute the youth justice system.
2 The establishment of methods of 'systems management' to ensure minimal intervention into the lives of the majority of young people and targeting of intensive services on those young people with the most established criminal careers.
3 The development of programmes of direct work with young people in community settings which both address the young people's offending behaviour and maintain the credibility of the public, police and courts in the method of work.
4 The development of routine means of monitoring the outcomes of the youth justice system to enable revisions in policy and practice when unintended consequences are identified.

This chapter will consider each of the elements individually, but it should be remembered that they cannot be disaggregated in practice and are essentially implemented simultaneously to be effective.

DEVELOPMENT OF LOCAL POLICIES

Research and policy analysis over the past twenty years has clearly established that the youth justice system is not a national system but a local system. Huge variations in practice between local units of the same services can be demonstrated at each stage of the system. Thus, for example, cautioning rates of police forces have continued to show wide variations between forces despite consistent attempts by the Home Office to reduce diversity (Giller and Tutt 1987). Variations in the rates at which local crown prosecutors 'retain' cases or divert them have been identified (Gelsthorpe and Giller 1990). The sentencing patterns of courts show such wide variations that the term 'justice by geography' is now widely accepted (Richardson 1989). And in social services the staff, finance and buildings committed to work with young offenders will vary enormously and are unrelated to the identified needs in the area, for example the provision of secure accommodation (Stewart and Tutt 1987).

It is clearly established that the law, most recently the Criminal Justice Act 1991, allows great latitude for local policy making. This being so it is essential that the local social services departments take a clear stance in pursuing negotiated agreed objectives with the police, crown prosecution service and courts. Social services must pursue the objective of diversion at all stages of the criminal justice system:

1 Diversion from crime through involvement in crime prevention.
2 Diversion from court through increased cautioning.
3 Diversion from custody through use of alternatives.

Diversion from crime

A number of local authorities, after publication of the Morgan Report (Morgan 1991), chose to take a lead role in community safety/crime prevention strategies. However, comparatively few of these initiatives have been led by social services, although it should be the experience and knowledge of social work that is the motive force. The Children Act 1989 places specific responsibilities on local authorities. These can be described as:

1 Having a responsibility to encourage children within their area not to commit criminal offences.
2 Having a responsibility to ensure that where state intervention is necessary it is limited to the minimum required to protect the child and the community.
3 Having to ensure that children's individual rights are protected at all times. This may mean financial assistance to ensure legal representation for the child.
4 Wherever possible, the child should be maintained within his or her own home with state or voluntary support. Removal from home should be a last resort.
5 All departments of central and local government should act corporately to provide services for children. There should not be contradictory services adopted by education, housing, social services, health services, leisure services or environmental services and employment services. For

example, children should not be exposed to adverse living conditions which are known to be detrimental merely because their parents have been evicted for non-payment of rent.

6   There should be a presumption at all times in favour of meeting the welfare needs of the child rather than incarcerating the child to protect the public. When children are responsible for criminal behaviour, wherever possible it should be dealt with outside the formal criminal justice system.

7   Central and local government have a responsibility to ensure that all staff working with children and young people and parents are supported by clear policies and procedures on factors important to the welfare of children, for example, access to health care, education, special needs assessment, protection from corporal punishment and dangerous drugs, including tobacco and alcohol.

8   There should be a clear commitment by central and local government to monitor, evaluate and report on the services to children to ensure policy objectives are being achieved and children are not being discriminated against on the basis of age, gender, sexuality or disability or any other aspect not of the individual's making.

Diversion from court

The most recent statistics on police cautioning illustrate a very substantial shift in practice over the past decade. Much of this shift has been achieved by the involvement of social workers in negotiations with police over who is suitable for caution. Moreover, marginal additions of service (for example, limited groupwork post-caution) have increased the likelihood of a second or third caution in a number of areas. The objective of the negotiation is to maximize the cautioning of juveniles and thereby remove them from the youth justice service. Table 8.2 shows the vast majority of police forces are now cautioning more than 70 per cent of the males under 17 years of age charged; the figure for females is even higher at over 90 per cent. Over the same period there has been a marked decline in the numbers of young people appearing in court from 81,000 to 24,600. The involvement of social workers in the negotiating of cautions appears to have contributed to achieving the objective of diverting young people from court.

Table 8.2 Percentage of males under 17 cautioned by the police by force area for 1981 and 1990

1981	%	1990
	− 87 −	Kent
	− 86 −	
	− 85 −	Dyfed-Powys
	− 84 −	Essex
	− 83 −	Devon & Cornwall, Hertfordshire
	− 82 −	
	− 81 −	Staffordshire
	− 80 −	Hampshire, West Mercia
	− 79 −	Cambridgeshire, Leicestershire, Warwickshire, Wiltshire
	− 78 −	Bedfordshire, Derbyshire, Gloucestershire, Norfolk, Northamptonshire, North Yorkshire
	− 77 −	Cheshire, Cleveland, Thames Valley, West Midlands
	− 76 −	Suffolk, West Yorkshire
	− 75 −	Cumbria, Humberside, Lincolnshire, Surrey, Sussex
	− 74 −	Metropolitan Police District
	− 73 −	Avon & Somerset, Lancashire, Gwent
	− 72 −	
	− 71 −	Dorset, Greater Manchester, Northumbria, Nottinghamshire
	− 70 −	Merseyside, South Wales
	− 69 −	North Wales
	− 68 −	South Yorkshire
	− 67 −	
	− 66 −	
	− 65 −	
Lincolnshire	− 64 −	
West Mercia, Essex	− 63 −	
Hampshire, Devon & Cornwall	− 62 −	
	− 61 −	
Suffolk	− 60 −	Durham
Surrey	− 59 −	
	− 58 −	
	− 57 −	
	− 56 −	
Nottinghamshire, Norfolk, Dyfed-Powys	− 55 −	
Bedfordshire, Cambridgeshire	− 54 −	
Sussex, Staffordshire	− 53 −	

Table 8.2 Continued

Thames Valley	– 52 –	
Northumbria, Dorset	– 51 –	
	– 50 –	
Northamptonshire, Hertfordshire	– 49 –	
North Wales	– 48 –	
Gloucestershire, West Midlands	– 47 –	
Wiltshire, Cumbria, Warwickshire	– 46 –	
Lancashire	– 45 –	
Kent, North Yorkshire, South Yorkshire	– 44 –	
Derbyshire, Leicestershire	– 43 –	
	– 42 –	
West Yorkshire, Avon & Somerset	– 41 –	
Gwent, Durham	– 40 –	
Cheshire, Metropolitan Police District	– 39 –	
Merseyside, Cleveland	– 38 –	
	– 37 –	
	– 36 –	
Humberside, Greater Manchester	– 35 –	
	– 34 –	
	– 33 –	
South Sales	– 32 –	
	– 31 –	
	– 30 –	
National Average 47 per cent		*National Average 75 per cent*

Source: *Criminal Statistics England and Wales 1981–1990*, London: Home Office.

Diversion from custody through use of alternatives

The methods employed within these alternatives are discussed later. In determining local policy social workers must take account of the significance of remands to custody as well as custodial sentences, and develop objectives to reduce both by maximizing opportunities for police bail, court bail and remands into local authority care.

SYSTEMS MANAGEMENT

It is the responsibility of social work to 'manage' the system, firstly because no other agency will; and secondly and more important, because the successful pursuit of clear objectives by management will ensure more positive and desirable outcomes for the user, and will prove cost effective for social services, since an unmanaged system will mean uncontrolled and inappropriate demands placed on social services. The flow chart (Figure 8.1) illustrates the system and points of intervention for social work.

The points at which social workers intervene in the system need to be clearly defined, the objective of their intervention should also be clearly defined, and their practice and outcome should be closely monitored. This is essential since social workers are not discrimination free. For example, the presentation of a pre-sentence report (social inquiry report) may contain elements of discriminatory practice. A recent study by Gelsthorpe (1992) states: 'Analysis of the content of 1152 pre-sentence social inquiry reports found the contrast between reports for males and females were much greater than between different ethnic groups.'

The main objective for social work intervention at all points of the youth justice system should be to achieve the least restrictive outcome for the young person compatible with the protection of that young person and the community.

DIRECT WORK WITH OFFENDERS

The thesis developed in this chapter is that delinquent behaviour results from specific situation determinants. The response from the police, courts and social agencies which make up the juvenile justice system will form a set of secondary situational determinants which can reinforce the delinquent image of the young person, thereby unintentionally maintaining the delinquent behaviour. By adopting a diversionary or minimal intervention stance, the juvenile justice system may reduce the likelihood of reinforcing the behaviour and therefore reduce the likelihood of recidivism.

The adoption of this approach has particular significance when assessing a juvenile offender for a treatment programme. Traditional treatment programmes have operated in generalized, if not grandiose, terms, very often omitting any comment or concentration on the actual offending behaviour. An alternative stance is to accept that offending behaviour is a result of specific situational determinants and rewarding after-effects. Such a stance leads to a treatment model in which a detailed analysis is made of the antecedents in the situation; the actual offending behaviour; and the outcomes, both in terms of actual rewards and believed outcomes on the part of the offender. Once this analysis has been undertaken a detailed 'attack' can be mounted on the behaviour in specific, strategic ways. For example, steps can be taken to reduce the possibility of the 'delinquent'

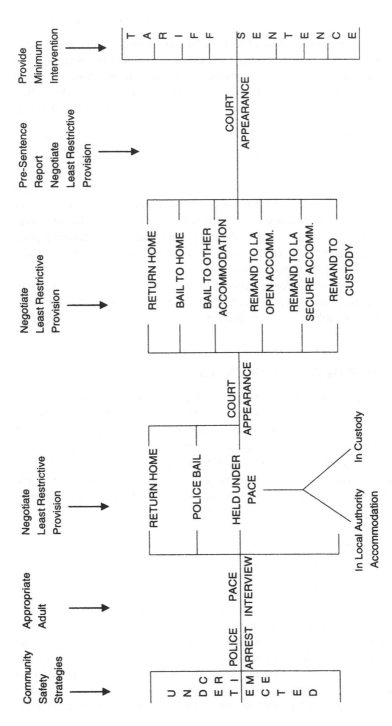

Figure 8.1 The social work role

situation being replicated, close surveillance may be provided to add a constraining determinant to the 'delinquent' situation, and new social skills which allow the offender to 'escape' without loss of status from delinquent situations can be taught. The actual and imagined rewards can be questioned publicly by the individual's peer group. There is nothing so effective for a male offender who believes his actions have led to him achieving status among his peers than to be confronted by them and told he is a 'wanker' or 'wally' for committing the offence. Denman (1983), working with males, has produced a handbook for practitioners, which attempts to develop an individualized assessment of offenders and a programme of treatment and objectives, as well as providing techniques for achieving these objectives. Denman's system is based on two guiding principles:

1 To discover, rather than attribute, 'reasons' or 'explanations' for a particular individual's specific delinquent action, in terms of phenomena at each different level, including situational phenomena.
2 To focus on private explanations and on individual accounts, which in effect means asking the offender.

Denman proposes a hierarchy of priorities for analysis and subsequent attack.

1 The behaviour and situation context – the specific details of the delinquent episode.
2 The reasoning behind the action – why did the offender decide to take part in this delinquent activity as opposed to other non-delinquent activities?
3 The general and more stable perceptions and philosophies held by the individual. The individual's account of specific phenomena (people, events, ideas, etc.) which arose in (2).
4 The past and present biographical events and situations which appear to be salient to (3).

Having constructed these priorities, Denman proposes using 'reasoning groupwork' based on knowledge from the social psychology of groups to:

1 Help the individual understand his own reasoning and belief system and how it influences behaviour.
2 Attack the beliefs which appear to be getting him into trouble.
3 Reinforce those beliefs which appear likely to stop him from getting into trouble.
4 Provide new beliefs which appear likely to stop him from getting into trouble.
5 Raise the importance he attaches to those beliefs which are likely to stop him from getting into trouble.

6 Lower the importance he attaches to those beliefs which appear to be getting him into trouble.
7 Raise and/or lower his certainty about outcomes as necessary.

Denman and others have implemented this programme with groups of male juvenile offenders. The programme is an interesting attempt to base a treatment model on the known evidence of situational determinants of crime. Moreover, it is an attempt to develop a treatment practice which also accepts minimal intervention. In Denman's programme, the 'professional' focuses attention solely on the individual's offending behaviour on the basis that state intervention is justified by that behaviour; other aspects of the offender's lifestyle – family, or belief structure – are ignored unless the offender declares them relevant to the offence. Such a degree of specificity strengthens both the position of the professional and the offender and would at least appear to have greater face validity than the generalized claims referred to earlier in this section.

MONITORING

Finally, since the problem of juvenile offending is now seen, in part at least, as being defined by the interaction between the individual juvenile and the youth justice system, and since the nature of its interaction influences the outcomes for the individual's delinquent career, social workers are being increasingly required to develop new methods with which to monitor the operation of the system. This is necessary because it is not easy to determine whether or not any one delinquent referred to an alternative programme would in fact be a 'candidate' for a custodial sentence did that programme not exist.

One of the possible solutions to this problem is the development of information systems which can monitor the workings of local youth justice systems and thereby evaluate the impact of changes in local policy and practice. Such a monitoring system works by separating out the characteristics of individual delinquents (in terms of their age, sex, race, area location, the offence and delinquent career) from official reaction to their behaviour, whether police, education, social or probation service or youth court reaction. Therefore it becomes possible to examine in detail total populations of delinquents and the ways in which official reactions to them are constructed and vary. Such a monitoring system seeks to answer two questions:

1 What are the essential characteristics of the local delinquent population and how do they vary over time?

2 What are the official responses to these juveniles and how are these responses constructed in terms of the interactions of local agencies? For example, does an increase in police cautioning affect the decisions made in the juvenile court?

For the purpose of system monitoring as well as evaluating the impact of the implementation of new services, the questions are reduced to:

1 What changes have occurred in the delinquent population?
2 What changes have occurred in official reactions which can be accounted for by: (a) changes in the delinquent population; (b) changes in the services provided?

The characteristics which illustrate these changes are assembled locally and then subjected to computer analysis (Social Information Systems 1983). Such monitoring allows key variables to be controlled. Thus, if a new service is introduced and then utilized by the court, is there a corresponding reduction in other 'target' sentences? If there is, can those two changes be causally linked? This is possible only if the juvenile population can be shown not to have changed substantially, nor the reactions changed, for example no increase in police cautioning. Only with these variables controlled can the service be deemed on target.

This approach to monitoring clearly reflects the developments in social work theory, since it attempts to tease out the significant factors which arise from the individual's behaviour and those which arise from the situation or reaction to that behaviour.

REFRENCES

Denman, G. (1983) *Intensive Intermediate Treatment with Juvenile Offenders*, Lancaster: Centre of Youth, Crime and Community, University of Lancaster.

Gelsthorpe, L. (1992) 'Social inquiry reports: race and gender considerations', in *Research Bulletin* no. 32, London: Home Office Research and Statistics Department.

Gelsthorpe, L. and Giller, H. (1990) 'More justice for juveniles', *Criminal Law Review*, March, 153–64.

Giller, H. and Tutt, N. (1987) 'Police cautioning of juveniles: does more mean better?', *Criminal Law Review*, March, 153–64.

Home Office (1992) *Race and the Criminal Justice System*, London: Home Office.

Morgan, J. (1991) *The Local Delivery of Crime Prevention through the Partnership Approach*, Home Office Standing Conference on Crime Prevention, London: HMSO.

Richardson, N. (1989 and 1990) *Justice by Geography* vols II and III, Knutsford: Social Information Systems.

Social Information Systems (1983), various reports on local juvenile justice systems, Knutsford: Social Information Systems.

Stewart, G. and Tutt, N. (1987) *Children in Custody*, London: Avebury.

Tutt, N. (ed.) (1978) *Alternative Strategies for Coping with Crime*, Oxford: Basil Blackwell.

9 Anti-racist social work

A black perspective

Shama Ahmed

It is a fact that racism operates at an ideological, structural, systemic and interpersonal level within contemporary British society. After the rebellions and uprisings of 1981 it became increasingly fashionable in some local government and social work circles to talk about the development of anti-racist policies and practices. But historically for black people (people of African, Caribbean and Asian origins) the struggles against racism in society and in social work did not commence at this juncture. Nor was anti-racist social work born in the closing years of the 1980s with the publication of books and articles bearing that label. The anti-racist struggles and campaigns of the 1960s in the factories and in the streets were authentic struggles of the black working class in Britain. During the 1970s and 1980s small numbers of black people began to occupy spaces not only in the factories but also in the town halls and professional bureaucracies. Black social workers realized how social inequalities are reproduced by welfare institutions.

Disproportionate numbers of black children are now in care, with less chance than white children of reunion with their parents (House of Commons Social Services Committee 1984; HMSO 1991). Welfare services for young offenders operate so inadequately that disproportionate numbers of black adolescents are in custodial establishments (Pitts *et al.* 1986; NACRO 1986 and 1988). Compulsory detention procedures for psychiatric treatment, especially involving use of police powers, are more common for the black community while voluntary admission procedures play a greater part for the white majority (Fernando 1988). Black elders rarely benefit from home help, meals on wheels, holidays and other support services designed for older people (Norman 1985; Patel 1990).

To understand how oppositional social work and forms of dissidence have developed it is important to sketch briefly the background and context within which social work with black communities initially emerged.

Questions of ethnic diversity surfaced quickly and sharply as social services workers in large conurbations began to face linguistic barriers, novel problems and new dilemmas. The ad hoc response of the local state was to employ one or two black workers. Although social services departments were slower than education departments to make use of section 11 of the 1966 Local Government Act, they began to rely on it. (Under this section central government funding is available for local authorities in order to meet the special needs of immigrants from the Commonwealth whose language and customs differ from the rest of the community.) The appointment of a few black workers was often the social services' only response and gesture towards a growing multiracial community. The use and misuse of this source of central government funding led to scandals and controversy. The full story of section 11 is beyond the scope of this chapter, but the underlying assumption of this approach is important to identify as it emphasized that problems facing black people were caused by the differentness of immigrants. Such an exclusive emphasis on cultural and linguistic differences tended to obscure the material condition of black people and their structural location in this society.

By the mid 1970s the general picture was one of limited or non-existent response by most local authorities to the question of racial inequality. In 1976 the Race Relations Act was passed. Whatever the limitations of the Act, it placed upon local authorities the duty to eliminate unlawful racial discrimination and promote equality of opportunity. The provision of social services to black communities was taken up at a national level by the Commission for Racial Equality which campaigned under the direction of its black social services officer for the development of a more relevant delivery of service for black children and families in the community.

Although social services paid little attention to the implications of the Race Relations Act for their various functions, black practitioners in the voluntary and statutory sector frequently spoke with a different voice, took risks and struggled against racism in their work. Resistance to racism in work with black children and black women are just two examples of their early efforts.

Black children began to enter local authority care in the 1960s. Work with them was dominated by the assimilationist ideology, which concentrated on transmitting a white identity to black children in care as superior and more desirable, an identity which was based on denial of their colour and race, and on self-hatred. Throughout the 1970s black practitioners, although few in number, challenged prevailing orthodoxies and racist institutional practices (Ahmed 1977a, 1978; Coombe 1975). It was not uncommon for black workers to be abused and labelled racists for challenging white mainstream practices.

Similarly, black women have been active since the 1970s in setting up autonomous refuges and safe places. For example, when Asian women facing male violence and mental distress went to white-run refuges they felt isolated and continued to be in psychological crisis. At the most stressful and critical time of their lives women found themselves in a completely alien environment and unable to benefit from affection and mutual support (Ahmed 1977b; Guru 1986; Wilson 1978). The activities of the Asian Women's Movement and the organisation of Women of Asian and African Descent bear witness to the battles black women were waging during the late 1970s (Bourne 1983; Bryan *et al.* 1985).

By the early 1980s racial politics were changing. Whatever the impact of the black rebellions of 1981 and 1983 in other fields, they seem to have acted as a mechanism for some local authorities to respond to the demands of their local black communities. There was promise of action to tackle racial discrimination in employment and service delivery, perhaps as a way of achieving some social peace. The black rebellions helped to shift the microscope from its initial focus on black minorities as *the* problem, to focus also on the majority society. White workers in the local state were expected to discover their personal racism and to learn to confront the racism of institutions in which they functioned.

Also in this period, the growth of National Front and racial violence involving large numbers of young white people forced many social workers to consider the implications of working with young Nazis on their case loads, notably in probation, intermediate treatment and residential settings. In 1981, following the murder of an Asian doctor by white youths, some of whom were in care, a social worker in a Midlands social services department wrote:

> There was not a day without some example of racist abuse. The residents had alternative words to the Specials' hit record *Ghost Town*, which began 'Do you remember the good old days before the wogs came?', followed by lines lampooning Caribbean and Asian physical characteristics, which contained vituperative obscenities. The chant 'Paki, Paki, Paki – out, out, out' was also very popular, as were racist jokes. Two children seriously believed Hitler was on the right lines and were anti-semitic as well as anti-black. This sort of behaviour is either ignored, or when staff do intervene they are dismissed as communists by the residents.
>
> (personal communication)

Another difference that the black unrest of 1981 made was the acceptance of racism by sections of the white left and the adoption of anti-racism as part of an agenda for municipal socialism. Until then many sections of the left had ignored racism and this neglect was reproduced in social work.

Even the (so-called) radical social work theorists seemed incapable of addressing themselves to race, for example *State Social Work and the Working Class* by Chris Jones (1983) and the influential collection of articles on radical social work edited by Roy Bailey and Mike Brake (1975, 1980) as well as the works of Paul Corrigan and Peter Leonard on Marxist social work (1978). In the main these theorists had a Eurocentric economic orientation and looked at class struggle in an orthodox way. They could not see race struggles as class struggles and seemed incapable of giving a real consideration to the structures of racial exploitation and racial oppression. In these ways the struggles of black people were written out of supposedly radical social work texts and so, for a black perspective, these texts were incomplete, orthodox and traditional in their ultimate impact on social work teaching and practice.

The same problems prevailed in white feminist theory and practice. Generalizations were based on the experiences of the dominant group and the terms of debate, direction, and worthwhileness of issues were set by white women. Black feminism and black women's political agendas were conspicuous by their absence. For example, it was not uncommon for work on the family, or male violence, to ignore black women's perspectives. As black feminists pointed out, the state had a different way of looking at black women. The ideology of the sanctity of family life which the state wishes to promote and the feminists want to question does not always apply to black communities. The state wishes to uphold white family life in its traditional form while at the same time undermining black family life (*Feminist Review* 1984).

Compared to progressive social work agencies, social work academics lagged behind in their experience of recognizing, let alone tackling racism. This group of people largely missed out on the anti-racist struggles, developments and gains made at the community and municipal level during the 1980s (Ahmed 1987). It took longer for white socialists and feminists to concede that social policy is both genderized as well as racialized (*Critical Social Policy* 1988).

Anti-racist social work requires a broad knowledge of state racism and an understanding of the plans of the state, including the political economy of racism. Practitioners need to grasp clearly the political context in which social work is located. They need to know in their minds and feel in their hearts the continuing relationship between underdevelopment for some and overdevelopment for others, colonization and the international movement of labour. Does this mean a constant indulgence in the rhetoric of racism? No, it is a question of awareness, of consciousness. It is above all a question of perspective. If the practitioner has brooded long and hard and seen the relationships between different parts of an unjust social structure and their effects on the individual, the perspective will come, and it will matter little whether the work is with small white children in a multiracial society or with black elders who are dying and bereaved. Anti-racist social work is informed by such a structural perspective and requires competence in countering cultural and institutional racism in assessment and intervention strategies. It also calls for a will to undertake non-institutional work and make connections with the wider anti-racist struggles in the community.

CULTURAL RACISM

Policy and action come out of the way we conceptualize things; concepts arise out of the material, historical and cultural matrix of society. In British society there is a hierarchy of cultures and those of racial minority groups are ranked very low indeed. If white British practitioners have had no help or preparation in raising their awareness of racism then there are bound to be problems with cultural explanations. It is not surprising, therefore, that references to black clients' cultures frequently reflect negative valuations rather than sensitivity. Even 'radical' practitioners who would not dream of pathologizing the culture of their poor white clients can fall into the racist trap of blaming minority group cultures. It is as though the black person spontaneously, by the very act of appearing on the scene, enters into a pre-existing framework of black cultures.

The abuses of cultural dimension in social work assessment and intervention are more fully discussed elsewhere (Ahmed 1986a). Perhaps to practitioners struggling to introduce into the work of their agencies a greater understanding of the culture of the service users, this coolness towards the cultural dimension may come as something of a surprise. However, the argument is not against better cultural understanding but against an over-reliance on cultural explanations which distract attention from significant emotional factors, as well as from structural factors such as gender, class and race. It is crucial to grasp the contradictions and tensions in culturally relevant work. Practitioners must recognize that social policy is always shot through with contradictory elements, as is the case with the Children Act 1989, and these have to be guarded against.

The Children Act 1989 is a significant political shift in social policy (Ahmed 1991a). For the first time in child care legislation, the local authorities will be under a duty to give due consideration, not only to religion, which has been part of child care law for many years, but also to three other important factors – a child's racial, ethnic and linguistic background (section 22 [5]). Seemingly, this will have major implications for social workers as it will be unlawful to ignore the race, culture, language and religion of children who are looked after by the statutory and voluntary institutions. However, multi-culturalism poses a number of theoretical and practice challenges which will have to be confronted.

First, multi-culturalism lacks a power analysis. It sees other cultures as valuable and interesting but the central reality of racism is either ignored, or racism is ascribed to the personal prejudices of a small number of ignorant, misguided or intolerant people. Most disconcertingly, it usually reflects a white view of black cultures as traditional, homogeneous, static and exotic. Culture is not seen as a continually changing process but as a relatively permanent characteristic of groups.

Second, multi-culturalism has been perverted by the arguments of the new right into a new form of racism, by converting cultural diversity into a deterministic theory of race. It has asserted the exclusivity of white British-ness and black people are not seen as part of the British nation. In the words of a National Front song, 'there ain't no black in the Union Jack'. Anyone not white is not British. They are the alien wedge and the enemy within. The intellectual organs of the new right such as the *Salisbury Review* have in the past decade of Thatcherism promoted a vulgar jingoistic nationalism in which the cultures, religions and lifestyles of Asian and African Caribbean people have been systematically disparaged and promoted as *so different* that they can threaten the social order (*Salisbury Review* 1982, 1983).

Third, multi-culturalism has done a disservice to black women's interests. Minority ethnic groups have come to be defined, as stated earlier, as being internally unified homogeneous entities with no class or gender differences or conflicts. For South Asian service users they have often come to be defined by religion only. Women's demands for freedom and equality have been seen in some arenas as clearly outside cultural traditions and therefore not re-garded as legitimate. By contrast, the most conservative traditions are considered the most authentic. This is a terrible trap for social workers who will need to develop a more sophisticated understanding of community and culture.

Minority ethnic groups are not internally unified entities without class and gender differences. Black women, in particular, often negotiate between a number of cultures. On the one hand, there can be the culture of the 'traditionalists' within the black communities. On the other hand, there is the culture of resistance to 'traditionalism'. Above all, there is the culture of racism of the dominant society. The culture of racism permeates all spec-trums of British society – the right and the left.

INSTITUTIONAL RACISM

Institutional racism is a limited but useful concept for illustrating how assumptions in the assessment and decision-making process can affect the provision, style and content of services. Key elements in recognizing institu-tional racism are the policies, practices and procedures and criteria of decision making which disproportionately disadvantage particular racial groups. Institutional racism is perpetuated even when there is a lack of intention to discriminate. Examples of institutional racism abound in the opportunity structures for training, jobs and access to services. A study of the internal arrangements of the London borough of Lambeth revealed a wide range of discriminatory practices through an analysis of traditional structures and policies. This study of the system shows quite clearly that the so-called 'colour blind' approach is discriminatory in its effects on different racial and cultural groups (Ouseley *et al.* 1983).

When considering access to services, the important point to note is that there can be concern both about *over-representation* as well as *under-repre- sentation* of minority ethnic groups in relation to their numbers and circumstances in the community. For instance, it is justifiable to examine whether there is a disproportionate number of black children in care. On the other hand, in many parts of the country Asian and African Caribbean offenders are usually under-represented in community based disposals and disproportionately over-represented in custodial sentences (NACRO 1986, 1988). We must also remember that the activities of social welfare agencies are not only concerned with social control functions but also with the provision of social support. Yet when it comes to social support some communities can suffer from too little intervention. For example there are widespread myths about the capacity of South Asian people and Chinese people to look after their own. Such ideas among care workers may under- estimate the needs of people for services.

Assessment of need and provision of services assumes a new importance under the Community Care and NHS act of 1990 (Dutt 1990; Johnson 1990). It took many years of agitation, struggles and pain to place race equality strategies on the agenda of local authorities, only to find that the system of local government as welfare state is being dismantled. In addition, mechan- isms such as contracting out largely favour the old established white voluntary sector which has either simply ignored, or significantly lagged behind in anti-racist work (Henry 1990).

Anti-racist social work expects answers to the following type of questions:

- Is the number of black children coming into care increasing? Why are they coming into care and are the reasons changing?
- Are the rates of registration of black people with physical disabilities the same as for the white population?
- Are aids and adaptations being given to black people at similar rates as white people and are they receiving community care services at the same level?
- What is the incidence of compulsory admissions under the Mental Health Act? Is is similar between all communities, black and white? What are the implications of high or low compulsory admission rates?

• Are black organizations receiving contracts for care? Are black carers receiving support?

It certainly cannot be assumed that just because an organization states its intention to offer equal opportunities to all, that will invariably be translated into practice. A system needs to be devised which can measure whether equal opportunities are, in fact, being offered. Yet record keeping and monitoring the delivery of social services to minority ethnic groups has been consistently resisted (Ahmed 1986b; Butt *et al.* 1991; Connelly 1985). This applies to traditional as well as to so-called progressive organizations such as feminist projects, and new services for people living with HIV and AIDS.

Of course, services are being ravaged and are in short supply and in the near future additional resources are likely to be limited. None the less, there is still a need to establish whether minority group members in social need stand an equal chance of receiving support. This raises issues of access to services as well as the style and content of services for those in the community who are at the bottom and have the least. Therefore, services must be appropriate at the point of delivery.

Anti-racist social work is also underpinned by another vital strand: the turning of cases into causes. Cases are alienated, disconnected and institutional; issues and causes are local, national and anti-institutional. Social workers see the operation of disadvantage and discrimination. They are strategically well placed to use it for the wider community. They must not confuse confidentiality with secrecy. The right of the black community to care for children in need is one example where concerted efforts to work closely with black parents, black councillors and other progressive forces in the community made some impact on provision of services (Ahmed 1980, 1986c; ABSWAP 1983). For far too long black child care issues were seen as professional matters when clearly they were political ones; and eventually agency centred, as well as community centred interventions were needed. Social workers working alone are in danger of repeatedly losing the power battles within their organizations. They need to recognize that working for change cannot be reduced to activity within office walls. They will need to broaden their tactics and link with the wider anti-racist struggles within the black communities.

Anti-racist social work must also recognize the contradictions and deficiencies of social work theories as well as their potential for analysis and action. There is space here only to demonstrate *some* problems with one of these theories – the psychodynamic treatment model – but this does not mean that other traditional social work theories are problem free (Ahmed 1991b). The difficulties are illustrated by the case of John Smith, 13 years old and charged jointly with five other white boys for causing damage to the seats of a school bus. All six youngsters made statements to the police admitting their guilt. The question to be addressed is: what difference do the class, gender and race of the client make? In so far as social work relies on the psychodynamic 'treatment' model, then to a large extent it tends, in practice, to divorce individuals from their social structural context and to locate problems firmly in the individual or in family pathology.

If John's situation is diagnostically understood on the basis of the psychodynamic treatment model, social workers will plan intervention to modify their client's personality. The worker's major tool in treatment will often be the use of self and the relationship with the client. The social workers will hope that the client's ego controls will be strengthened by building up his self-esteem, expressing love and concern and providing an example of benevolent authority perhaps through a supervision order. Alternatively, John's family group may become the target of intervention and some modifications of interaction patterns and attitudes within the family may become the treatment goal. This belief system can lead to a disproportionate amount of consideration being given to John as an individual and little to the wider social system with which he interacts. It ignores the institutionalized class bias in the processing of young offenders. Implicitly and sometimes explicitly mothers may be blamed. In the case of white mothers the blame is likely to be individualized but black mothers are blamed collectively. Negative images of black family life have crept into social work and social policy analysis. The African Caribbean family is often seen as a tangle of pathology, virtually non-existent as a unit or rapidly falling apart, with mothers being seen as too strong and over-committed to wage earning. On the other hand, the Asian family is seen as problematic because the mother's position is considered weak and uninfluential (Scarman Report 1981; Ahmed *et al.* 1986a).

As behaviour in the psychodynamic treatment model is seen as unconsciously motivated, and rule breaking is interpreted as a symptom of underlying emotional needs, particular difficulties in personal relationships and personality problems may well be identified. Eurocentric ideas of 'normality' and 'pathology' are influential. Narrow concepts of good child-rearing patterns, bonding processes, and what constitutes rejection and disruption often prevail. Individuals who are raised in extended families in the most formative years of their lives and who may have had many people to relate to can be seen as lacking in capacity for strong relationships. Many of us from the black communities would fail this kind of normality test.

Had the case concerned a white girl (Jane Smith, not John Smith) another kind of normality test might operate whereby sex role expectations may play their part. After all, girls who like to roam the streets freely as boys do, or to climb trees and participate in even mildly 'aggressive' or 'assertive' behaviour are nicknamed tomboys in white British cultures. So a group of white girls who might have ripped the seats of a bus would be seen as very troublesome indeed. Jane's actions may not only be seen as 'pathological', they may also be compounded with moral overtones. Jane may be seen as 'at risk', 'in moral danger', 'beyond parental control'. These have been grounds for obtaining care orders – a harsher disposal than community-based options.

What if the case had concerned black children? What kinds of disposals could be expected? It is a fact that even the psychodynamically oriented white practitioners have frequently taken flight from working with black clients. They have argued that when supervision orders are recommended they are expected to form a relationship with the client. However, because they often experience communication problems with black defendants they see little point in recommending therapeutic or other community-based disposals. This approach invariably results in harsher outcomes for black offenders (Pitts *et al.* 1986).

The important point is to recognize that social work theory as well as social work action are both genderized as well as racialized. There are problems with anti-racist strategies if they are seen in isolation from other disadvantages and oppressions. It is far too readily assumed that new social movements are essentially progressive. Yet, the politics of anti-racism has shown a limited capacity to tackle the institutionalized sexism of white agencies and the sexism of black cultures. It is apparent that anti-racism itself cannot be a complete philosophy. Anti-racism has to be class conscious. It has to be gender conscious. It should not be detached from the politics of other oppressions such as sexuality and disability. Society is clearly divided not only by race, but also by gender and class, but theorizing about race, gender and class together has not often taken place. The issue for anti-racist social work is to bring it together in both theory and practice.

It will be obvious by now that anti-racist work is rooted in a structural analysis of society and social work. It requires the capacity to work at different levels and requires many different types of skills and abilities. Such an analysis can lead to interventions which can be agency centred (e. g. changing discriminatory policies), or community centred (supporting campaigns for better resources), or individual centred (supporting individuals and working with mental distress and unhappiness). This form of work requires skills and understanding of collaborative as well as conflict methods. Competence in individual work, groupwork and community work as well as organizational change is relevant.

The work of black practitioners with black children and black women referred to in the introductory sections of this chapter are two examples where a combination of methods has been required. Practitioners have needed theories for black clients' emotional well being, as well as skills in individual and groupwork, for example working with individual children who have spoiled identities, and working in groups with children and adults to discover collectively the roots of oppression. They have also been more than prepared to do political work at a community campaigning level (Ahmed 1980, 1986c; Ahmad 1990; Maxime 1986). This style of work has often bridged traditional polarizations between community work and casework. Those who hanker for a return to social work's conservative roots have missed the meaning of anti-racist social work.

Whatever the method of social work, anti-racist practice is grounded in a social action perspective and should include the following:

Developing a critical consciousness is an ability to analyse social work situations in social and political terms, understanding the political connections, local and global relationships and change and development within organizations and communities.

Accountability means that the question of power cannot be ducked; anti-racist social workers should always try to shift it downwards towards service users.

Empowerment means working out possibilities of change with affected people themselves and facilitating political organization amongst service users.

Knowing the community, its strengths and the difficulties it faces; being involved in its struggles.

Knowing the agency is to be well informed about how policies are developed and to challenge inequalities. Developing influencing skills and strategies for organizational change.

Collective working means promoting and supporting practices which help in building a supportive culture wherever possible. Avoiding adventurism and isolationism; working towards organizational democracy.

Expert testimony entails organizing professional comment on specific issues, for example supporting lesbian mothers in custody cases.

This is not an exhaustive list, but some critical triggers for what is often required.

Anti-racist work has been attacked not only by the right, who are implacably opposed to any form of affirmative action at collective, or national and local state level, but its validity has also been questioned by black academics, who have sometimes presented it as simply the bureaucratization of oppression (Gilroy 1987a and b). More fundamentally, there are those who would challenge the whole notion of race equality strategies within a highly class-stratified society (Sivanandan 1985, 1991).

The relationship between class and race is not a new debate, it has raged at least since the beginning of this century (Robinson 1983). Many black radicals saw racial divisions as the most important cleavage in metropolitan societies. They were not always prepared to subsume race under class. The key points in their analysis were that there is a racial division of labour even when black people are employed. The working class in white metropolitan societies is racially segmented and there is an aristocracy of labour. There are classes within classes and black people are overwhelmingly in the lowest reaches of the economy. In post-imperial Britain most profit has been extracted from black workers, especially black women (Bryan *et al.* 1985). Black workers are exploited by the bosses and oppressed by fellow workers. To summarize in Toney Ottey's phrase, 'It may be that blacks are in the same boat as poor whites; but we are on different decks' (Ottey 1978).

The conceptions 'equality of opportunity', 'racial equality', 'anti-racism' and 'black perspectives', and the strategies which are proposed, must indeed be subjected to critical evaluation. They are not self-sufficient positions. All these notions are fundamentally limited in their impact. They are a coat of paint. They do not have the power to transform society. Anti-racist social work does not embody an epic version of change. But it cannot wait for the complete dismantling of Britain's stratified and unjust society. The point is that social work needs to understand that some people are exploited and oppressed because of their class position, some are exploited and oppressed because of class and gender, and some are exploited and oppressed because of class, race *and* gender. To this can be added further oppression and discrimination which is based on disability, ageism, sexuality and so on. Hence the notion of multiple oppressions must be taken seriously in social work (Baxter *et al.* 1990; Begum 1992).

Anti-racist social workers understand only too well that legal action, new laws and better cultural understanding will not eradicate racism, sexism, disablism or poverty. There is no cause for complacency. Racism keeps changing forms and requires new combative strategies. The adoption of anti-racist policy itself can also be a way of managing and neutralizing black resistance at local and national levels. Therefore, anti-racist practice should be critical practice.

REFERENCES

ABSWAP (1983) *Black Children in Care, Evidence to the House of Commons Social Services Committee*, London: Association of Black Social Workers and Allied Professions.

Ahmad, B. (1990) *Black Perspectives in Social Work*, Birmingham: Venture Press.

Ahmed, S. (1977a) 'Midland mother loses fight for children', *The West Indian World*, 23 December.

Ahmed, S. (1977b) 'Sahaara, Asian women's residential centre', unpublished discussion paper, Wolverhampton Council for Community Relations.

Ahmed, S. (1978) 'Children in care: the racial dimension in social work assessment', *Working with Asian Young People*, National Association for Asian Youth.

Ahmed, S. (1980) 'Selling fostering to the black community', *Community Care*, 6 March, 20–22.

Ahmed, S. (1986a) 'Cultural racism in work with Asian women and girls', in S. Ahmed, J. Cheetham and J. Small (eds) *Social Work with Black Children and their Families*, London: Batsford.

Ahmed, S. (1986b) 'Ethnic record keeping: questions and answers', in V. Coombe and A. Little (eds) *Race and Social Work*, London: Tavistock.

Ahmed S. (1986c) 'Setting up a community foster action group', in V. Coombe and A. Little (eds) *Race and Social Work*, London: Tavistock.

Ahmed, S. (1987) 'Let's break through the barriers to equality', *Community Care*, 29 October, *Inside* supplement.

Ahmed, S. (1991a) 'Routing out racism', *Community Care*, 27 June, 16–18.

Ahmed, S. (1991b) 'Developing anti-racist social work education practice', in CCETSW, *Setting the Context for Change*, London: CCETSW.

Bailey, R. and Brake, M. (1975) *Radical Social Work*, London: Edward Arnold.

Bailey, R. and Brake, M. (1980) *Radical Social Work and Practice*, London: Edward Arnold.

Baxter, C., Poonia, K., Ward, L. and Nadirshaw, Z. (1990) *Double Discrimination: Issues and Services for People with Learning Difficulties from Black and Ethnic Minority Communities*, London: Kings Fund Centre.

Begum, N. (1992) *Different Lives, Same Rights*, Waltham Forest: Race Relations Unit.

Bourne, J. (1983) 'Towards an anti-racist feminism', *Race and Class*, Summer, 1–22.

Bryan, B., Dadzie, S. and Scafe, S. (1985) *The Heart of the Race: Black Women's Lives in Britain*, London: Virago.

Butt, J., Gorbach, P. and Ahmad, B. (1991) *Equally Fair?*, London: Race Equality Unit.

Connelly, N. (1985) *Social Services Departments and Race: A Discussion Paper*, London: Policy Studies Institute.

Coombe, V. (1975) *Fostering Black Children*, London: Commission for Racial Equality.

Corrigan, P. and Leonard, P. (1978) *Social Work Practice Under Capitalism: A Marxist Approach*, London: Macmillan.

Critical Social Policy (1988) 'Racism, anti-racism and the editorial collective', issue 21, 4–7.

Dutt, R. (ed.) (1990) *Black Community and Community Care*, London: NISW Race Equality Unit.

132   *Practising social work*

Feminist Review (1984) *Many Voices One Chant: Black Feminist Perspectives*, Autumn.

Fernando, S. (1988) *Race and Culture in Psychiatry*, Beckenham: Croom Helm.

Gilroy, P. (1987a) *Problems in Anti-Racist Strategy*, London: The Runnymede Trust.

Gilroy, P. (1987b) *There Ain't No Black in The Union Jack*, London: Hutchinson.

Guru, S. (1986) 'An Asian women's refuge', in S. Ahmed, J. Cheetham and J. Small (eds) *Social Work with Black Children and their Families*, London: Batsford.

Henry, I. (1990) 'To be forewarned is to be forearmed – the Birmingham experience', in L. Johnson (ed.) *Contracts for Care*, London: National Council for Voluntary Organizations.

House of Commons Social Services Committee (1984) *Children in Care* vol. 1, London: HMSO.

HMSO (1991) *Patterns and Outcomes in Child Placement*, London: HMSO.

Johnson, L. (1990) *Contracts for Care*, London: National Council for Voluntary Organizations.

Jones, C. (1983) *State Social Work and the Working Class*, London: Macmillan.

Maxime, J. E. (1986) 'Some psychological models of black self concept', in S. Ahmed, J. Cheetham and J. Small (eds) *Social Work with Black Children and their Families*, London: Batsford.

National Association for the Care and Resettlement of Offenders (NACRO) (1986) *Black People and the Criminal Justice System*, London: NACRO.

National Association for the Care and Resettlement of Offenders (NACRO) (1988) *Some Facts and Figures in the Criminal Justice System*, London: NACRO.

Norman, A. (1985) *Triple Jeopardy: Growing Old in a Second Homeland*, London: Centre for Policy on Ageing.

Ottey, T. (1978) quoted in C. Cross, *Ethnic Minorities in the Inner City*, London: Commission for Racial Equality.

Ouseley, H., Silverstone, D. and Prashar, U. (1983) *The System*, London: The Runnymede Trust.

Patel, N. (1990) *A 'Race' Against Time?*, London: The Runnymede Trust.

Pitts, J., Sowa, T., Taylor, A. and Whyte, L. (1986) 'Developing an anti-racist intermediate treatment', in S. Ahmed, J. Cheetham and J. Small (eds) *Social Work with Black Children and their Families*, London: Batsford.

Robinson, C. J. (1983) *Black Marxism*, London: Zed Press.

Salisbury Review, Autumn 1982, Summer 1983.

Scarman, Lord (1981) *The Scarman Report: The Brixton Disorders*, Harmondsworth: Penguin.

Sivanandan, A. (1985) 'RAT and the degradation of black struggle', *Race and Class*, Spring, no. 4, 1–33.

Sivanandan, A. (1991) 'Black struggles against racism' in CCETSW, *Setting the Context for Change*, London: CCETSW.

Wilson, A. (1978) *Finding a Voice: Asian Women in Britain*, London: Virago.

FURTHER READING

Ahmad, Arshi (1990) *Practice with Care*, London: NISW Race Equality Unit.

CCETSW (1991) *One Small Step Towards Racial Justice*, London: CCETSW.

Connelly, N. (1990) *Between Apathy and Outrage: Voluntary Organizations in Multiracial Britain*, London: Policy Studies Institute.

hooks, bell. (1989) *Talking Back: Thinking Feminist – Thinking Black*, London: Sheba Feminist Publishers.

Institute of Race Relations (1982) *Roots of Racism*, London: IRR.

Sivanandan, A. (1982) *A Different Hunger: Writings on Black Resistance*, London: Pluto Press.

10 Crisis intervention: changing perspectives

Kieran O'Hagan

The importance of crisis intervention as a method of professional practice is manifest in the frequency with which it is used, and the diversity of clients and crisis situations to which it is applied. Here is a random selection of crises which necessitate intervention; the professional, or ethical, or legal obligations to intervene should be apparent:

1 A woman is battered by her cohabitee. She and her terrified pre-school children desperately seek refuge.
2 A Pakistani child, aged 11, subjected to persistent racist bullying over a long period of time, bursts into tears during a school lesson. He is uncontrollable and the parents and the school staff feel helpless.
3 An elderly confused man accidentally sets his house on fire. The neighbours rescue him; they are also elderly. They are in a state of fear and panic; he has subjected them to danger before, and they are certain he will do so again. They demand his removal, as does a GP and psychiatrist.
4 A reconstituted family erupts in violence perpetrated by the stepfather against his teenage stepdaughter. He accuses her of deliberately sabotaging the family's attempts to achieve harmony and stability, and demands that she leaves.
5 Two teenage children and their mother watch helplessly as three hooded men break into their home and murder the father in a sectarian attack.
6 A man learns that he is HIV positive, through infection by his wife. She was infected through extramarital affairs which he knew nothing about.
7 A Nigerian woman arrives in Britain, to be reunited with her husband. She speaks very little English. She is detained by immigration officers, who allege irregularities in her passpost and visa. She is told (unofficially) to 'get back to where she belongs'. Meanwhile, she is transported to a 'processing' centre, and denied access to her husband. She is extremely frightened, and dwells upon many unpleasant thoughts about what might happen to her.
8 A man leaves his home, job, and spouse after a twenty-year period. He

soon finds that he cannot cope with the changes he has brought upon himself. Nor does he feel that he can return. His mental health rapidly deteriorates. He attempts to kill himself.

9 A woman agrees to her child being medically examined because of the suspicion that her cohabitee has sexually abused the child. The woman is deeply distressed by the allegation, but accepts that the examination is in everyone's interest, particularly the child's. However, she is totally unprepared for the detail of the examination. She watches with increasing horror and disgust as the male paediatrician systematically examines the child's genitals. The woman is traumatized for some days after, and incapable of co-operating with the agencies.

10 A woman's financial hardship increases gradually over a six-month perioid after her husband abruptly leaves her. She feels more isolated and stigmatized in a locality where she has no roots, far distant from parents and former social contacts. The quality of care she provides for her three children, aged 8, 6 and 3, deteriorates. She is visited by a social worker, a health visitor and an educational welfare officer, all of whom express concern. They offer help and support, but she perceives their efforts as further stigmatizing her, and as holding her responsible for the predicament in which she now finds herself. She is visited by a DSS officer who presses her about the whereabouts of her husband for the purpose of extracting maintenance from him. She is made to feel like a criminal harbouring her husband; the officer concerned is indifferent to her financial plight. She receives a letter from the DSS saying that they have been overpaying her slightly and that she must pay them back or do with less than her existing weekly allowance. She becomes hysterical, and runs out of her home, leaving her three children. She is found wandering on the motorway, and is taken to a police station.

Before looking at the task of defining crisis, an important point should be made in the light of these examples. They are all complex and difficult cases. Each one of them poses numerous differing and related challenges. For example, the crisis of the bullied Pakistani child may reveal a host of social, economic, and cultural challenges, some of which can be dealt with over a period of time by methods other than crisis intervention, such as community work, report writing and advocacy, groupwork, establishing better liaison with police and education, and so on. These tasks do not necessitate crisis intervention; the child's suffering and uncontrollable weeping, as a consequence of persistent racist bullying, does necessitate immediate crisis intervention. Very often in crisis literature, much space is taken up in describing the application of approaches, skills and techniques which are standard tools in a variety of social work methods, for example listening, pacing, empathizing, and so on. This chapter will not repeat this list. It will trace the development of crisis intervention, highlight some of its strengths and weaknesses in application, and suggest principles and foundations for a modern, effective crisis intervention service.

DEFINITION OF CRISIS

Some prominent crisis pioneers may contest the view that all of these cases are crises. Caplan (1961, 1964) defined a crisis in terms of clearly identifiable processes, developing over a period of weeks, and leading to a climactic (crisis) point. The experiences may be so overwhelming and threatening that the individual cannot cope within their existing resources. Pittman (1973) makes a distinction between 'crisis' and 'emergency':

> Crisis is a more subtle concept: it may occur without all the turmoil of a subjective emergency state. It involves a process of systems change, is far more objective, and is not something to be relieved but something to be solved.
>
> (p.99).

Wright (1991) differentiates between stress and crisis: 'Stress and crisis are different. A stressful event produces anxiety and tension. A crisis disturbs old established patterns of responding' (p. 23).

Parad and Caplan (1965) used systems theory language to define crisis: 'A crisis is a period of disequilibrium overpowering the individual's homeostatic mechanisms' (p. 56).

Langsley *et al.* (1968) gave up trying to define crisis, yet their concluding remarks are helpful: '... crisis theory has defined the crisis as the hazardous event (stress) and the subsequent reaction to that event' (p. 156).

Thompson (1991) clarifies: 'the subjective dimension is primary, for an event not perceived as a crisis will not be experienced as a crisis' (p. 11).

O'Hagan (1986) suggests that the most relevant meaning of crisis for social workers lies within the Greek and Chinese origins of the word. 'Crisis' derives from the Greek *krisis*, meaning decision making; the Chinese represent the word with symbols denoting danger and opportunity. Thus crisis is a time for decision making in a situation presenting danger and opportunity.

All of these attempts to define are interesting, but it's important to avoid becoming too preoccupied with definitions. Emphasis upon subjective experiences is sensible. One may say that the crises listed in the opening of this chapter do not all fall within classical crisis theory and definition, but who would deny any of those individuals the right to say that they are experiencing crises of major proportions?

THE ORIGINS AND DEVELOPMENT OF CRISIS INTERVENTION

The origins of crisis intervention owe little to such diversity. The focus of the crisis pioneers was extremely narrow in comparison with the crisis work undertaken by social workers today. The pioneers of crisis intervention were predominantly American psychiatrists in the 1940s and 1950s. They coined the phrase 'crisis intervention', and developed the method. Their pioneering work centred mainly upon the mental health crises of their patients in their clinics and psychiatric hospitals, and in later years upon the crises which the mental condition of those patients generated among their families. The following is a very brief summary of some contributions made to crisis theory and practice and its development over five decades.

Lindemann's (1944) 'Symptomatology and management of acute grief' has long been recognized as the first major crisis research. He studied the mourning reactions of people whose relatives had been killed in a Boston night club fire disaster. His detailed, systematic observations provided a psychodynamic theoretical framework which was developed by Caplan (1961, 1964). Caplan produced a unified theory of crisis which became central to his conceptual model of primary prevention in mental health. Although Caplan's theory, like Lindemann's, evolved from psychoanalytical concepts, he was aware of the possibility that family and socio-cultural factors could have a bearing on the outcome of crisis. His analysis of crisis processes indicates the application of some basic concepts in systems theory.

Rapoport (1971) projected crisis intervention as a mode of brief treatment, less time consuming, and more effective than the classical psychoanalytical model. Yet her contribution depends heavily upon psychoanalytical concepts, as well as traditional casework methods (she was the only social worker amongst the pioneers), and upon the psychodynamic developmental life crises formulated by Erikson (1965). Rapoport wrote:

> Crisis theory, insofar as it requires an understanding of the individual, needs to be anchored in personality theory. Psychoanalytical theory, first as it developed into a theory of the neuroses and in its latter evolution into a theory of personality... still seems to serve as the most useful base because of the comprehensiveness of the phenomena described. All developments in ego psychology are of great significance in crisis theory.
> (p.87).

Aguilera and Messick (1980) provided a model of assessment for crisis situations, and an intervention model. Both are firmly based upon systems theory's concept of homeostasis. Langsley (1968) consolidated the influence of systems theory on the development of crisis theory. Systems theory concepts underpin the intervention model that he and his colleagues devised, specifically for mental health crises. The research and practice of Langsley and colleagues (1971) coincided with the rapid development of family therapy. The foundations of family crisis intervention were then laid from a synthesis of strategies developed in crisis intervention and family therapy; the latter would soon emerge as the dominant influence in family crisis intervention. Bott (1976) and Scott (1974) widened the focus still further. They defined mental health crisis within the context of patient, family, hospital and community, and within the historical, social and political processes which shaped the perceptions of mental illness, and dictated the nature of psychiatric provision in general.

O'Hagan (1984, 1986) reviewed literature and research on crisis intervention in the light of his own experiences as a generic social worker. He found it seriously flawed in its lack of an adequate ethical foundation. He emphasized the conflictual nature of most crises, and explored the ethical dilemmas arising from such conflict. O'Hagan evolved a crisis theory and intervention strategy from systems theory concepts and family theory techniques. This theory and strategy can be applied in coping with many of the harsh realities of crisis situations in which British social workers often find themselves, for example crises of threat and violence; crises in which families and neighbours are clamouring for the removal of a child at risk, an elderly confused person, a mentally ill family member, a wayward delinquent.

Eisler and Hersen (1973) and more recently, Thompson (1991) advocate a behaviourist approach to crises, underpinned by social learning theory. 'Reinforcement' and 'goal setting' are key concepts in empowering people in crisis by facilitating their learning of more effective coping skills: 'The ultimate goal of any counsellor dealing with clients in crisis is to teach new and better coping skills' (Thompson 1991: 25). Reinforcement for this purpose has to be sufficient, immediate and consistent. Thompson additionally argues for an existential perspective, 'with its emphasis on the interplay of subjective and objective factors, unpredictability and uncertainty, and the need to take positive control of one's life' (p. 17).

RELEVANCE AND LIMITATIONS WITHIN THE CRISIS HERITAGE

This legacy and development in crisis work is impressive. Much of it influences current approaches to crises. For example, the importance of a theoretical underpinning (whichever one may choose) is accepted as crucial in present-day training for crisis work. Many of the principles and techniques which evolved from the work of the pioneers are still regarded as necessary for approaching the crisis with the right attitude, and effective for speedily relieving individuals in crisis from the pain and danger to which they are often exposed.

The early pioneers were, however, unaffected by issues such as gender and race. They were unaware of how such issues manifested themselves in crisis processes and crisis eruption (O'Hagan 1991). Concepts such as institutional racism and sexism and structural oppression and deprivation (Dominelli 1988; Davis 1991) had no place either in their theoretical frameworks or in their intervention models. Later contributors to the crisis legacy did become aware of these concepts. Thompson (1991) comments:

> ... traditional crisis theory can be criticised for adopting a predominantly white, middle class, male perspective on a range of issues which relate very closely to structured inequalities and the oppressive social divisions which stack the odds against certain groups in society.
>
> (p. 15)

O'Hagan (1989, 1992) explores what he calls the 'endemic' and 'institutionalized' abuse of women perpetrated unwittingly by many child care organizations in child protection crises generally, and in the crises of child sexual abuse in particular. Wright (1991) gives examples of the damaging sexist attitudes of well meaning male friends and relatives of women stricken by the crises generated by the sudden deaths of their husbands or children. Though not writing about any aspect of crisis or crisis intervention, Currer (1991) none the less demonstrates how racism and its associated insensitivity amongst professionals responding to Pathan women engaging in Ramadan fasting during pregnancy may actually generate crises where none previously existed!

HOW STRUCTURAL OPPRESSION AND ISSUES AROUND GENDER MAY INFLUENCE CRISES

Crisis intervention is no different from any other discipline in that its proper development, relevance and usefulness depend upon periodical critical scrutiny. Public welfare services in general have been found wanting in their lack of awareness about issues such as race, gender and structural inequalities. The continuing importance and effectiveness of crisis intervention depends fundamentally upon its advocates ensuring that such issues positively influence their attitudes as much as their actions. This point is more clearly understood if we consider a possible scenario for one of the cases mentioned in the opening pages, that of the woman found wandering on the motorway (case no. 10). Let us imagine that when you and your colleague get to the police station, the desk sergeant welcomes you and talks about the woman 'flipping her lid' because 'her husband walked out on her'. Another officer suggests 'she needs to see a psychiatrist'. The woman is in no mood to talk to you. She is frightened and repeatedly fluctuates between prolonged weeping and angry emotional outbursts. She has already been compelled to talk ceaselessly about herself to the patrol officers who picked her up, and to the police surgeon who declared that she wasn't in need of psychiatric help. She has repeatedly asked officers to take her back to her home, or to allow her to leave. The officers have persuaded her to stay until you and your colleague have arrived.

The police, unwittingly, may have worsened this crisis considerably. The flight in which the woman engaged – a common and natural response – may have been an effective coping mechanism for surviving the latest calamity of the letter from the DSS. At the very least, it can be an unmistakable cry for help. (It's not exactly desirable though for the safety and mental health of the children, an issue warranting much time and attention beyond the brief of this chapter.) But now this woman has to cope with the additional problems of being picked up by the police, detained in a police station, and subjected to repeated questioning stemming from blatant discriminatory (sexist, anti-disability) stereotyping attitudes. The consequences are likely to further undermine her self-identity, her confidence and competence.

The speediest accompanied return to her children and to her role as mother and protector is the first priority in this case. (Some workers may dash to the children first, an action likely to be perceived by the woman as an extension of the undermining which was carried out in the police station.) At home, when time and situation permit, when she thinks and feels that it is beneficial and desirable for her to reflect, then validating her crisis is the next priority. This does not mean persuading her that she has done the right thing; she most likely realizes she hasn't. It means helping her to understand that there is a link between (1) the various forms of poverty and stigma to which she has been exposed, and (2) her increasing fear and anxiety which led inevitably to a climactic eruption. This will be a significant step forward in convincing her that she is neither 'mad' nor 'bad'. Such self-perceptions easily take root in the minds of clients, particularly in those at the centre of mental health and child abuse crises.

Systems theory, social learning theory, and psychodynamic and developmental theories could all make some contribution towards enlightening client and worker about the client's internal state and about her rapidly deteriorating situation. But none of these theoretical orientations directly addresses the contributory factors of structural oppression and stigma, institutionalized sexism, and anti-disability attitudes (e. g. ridicule and isolation of the individual labelled as disabled). Other more recent theoretical orientations mentioned in this chapter certainly do address these factors, particularly

Davis (1991). (See also Popay 1991 for a perceptive structural analysis most relevant to the case in question.)

FOUNDATIONS OF A MODERN CRISIS INTERVENTION SERVICE

The foundations of a modern effective crisis intervention service have four major components: a sound ethical base, appropriate conceptual and/or theoretical frameworks, a sufficient level of self awareness within the professionals dealing with crises, and a repertoire of skills and techniques. Each of these components will be enhanced in terms of importance and effectiveness if it combines many of the achievements of the crisis pioneers with an increased awareness of the wider cultural, structural and institutional context of crises. The four components need to be explained in more detail.

1 A sound ethical base

Ethical considerations in social work generally have been extremely narrow and limiting in respect of enlightening workers about the nature of the dilemmas they often face. The ethical challenge in crisis intervention is unmistakably complex and formidable. It cannot be surmounted merely by the right 'ethical' attitude. It often requires *action* in which ethically sound attitudes are clearly manifest. The ethical base of crisis intervention requires the following:

(a) A system of values which are resolutely opposed to discrimination in all its various forms, that is discrimination because of race, religion, age, gender, disability, sexual orientation, and so on. The 'resolution' and the 'opposition' will often necessitate honesty and courage on the part of the worker: for example, to confront a police officer, a psychiatrist, or a paediatrician, about actions or attitudes that are clearly exacerbating the client's predicament.

(b) Knowledge and experience: there is a fundamental ethical obligation for workers engaged in crisis intervention to be reasonably knowledgeable, experienced and confident in facing crises. There is an even greater ethical responsibility upon managers to ensure that front-line workers have every opportunity to acquire knowledge, experience and confidence· in all aspects of crisis work. For example, it is highly unethical to send a newly qualified, unapproved social worker, alone, to investigate a complex mental health crisis. It is also highly unethical on the part of a worker who embarks upon a crisis, fully conscious of her lack of knowledge, and as fearful as she is certain that she will provide the worst possible service to the client. Again, great honesty and courage are needed on the part of both front-line workers and managers to face up to the clearly unethical nature of such actions, and to avoid them.

(c) Appropriate use of power and control on behalf of clients: this may be necessary in upholding the rights of clients; conversely, it may be necessary in getting crisis participants to surrender what they perceive to be their rights; for example, a father may believe that the extreme and damaging authority he exercises over his wife or daughter is his right. He may be influenced or persuaded to think otherwise; if not, power and control are legitimate ethical tools to ensure that basic rights of the mother and daughter are established (wife battering and child sexual abuse are probably the most common crises in which professionals are ethically justified in using power and control to protect the child/woman from such abuses).

(d) Adequate resources, and the constant reappraisal of existing resources by crisis workers and their managers to ensure that they remain adequate. The crises of child sexual abuse have highlighted the ethical nature of the resources issue: it is unethical to compulsorily remove children from the risk of sexual abuse if the authority has not satisfactory alternative care and protection to offer the child; similarly with any other clients in crisis, it is unethical to intervene if the workers/agencies involved do not have the resources (personnel, expertise, finance, accommodation, etc.) to ensure the likelihood of a successful intervention.

2   Conceptual and/or theoretical frameworks

It is vital for professionals responsible for crisis intervention to have a sound theoretical base underpinning their methods. The conceptual and/or theoretical frameworks which professionals adopt should be flexible. They should facilitate understanding of the structural factors causing, contributing to, and sustaining the crisis, for example poverty, stigma or organizational and/or cultural rigidity. All theory should provide a predictive facility; crisis theory should enable the worker to predict the direction and outcome of crisis processes, and the impact of the worker's attempt to intervene.

3   Self-exploration

It is crucial for workers to be aware of the major sources of challenge to them personally, in the crisis situation. These challenges could arise from the most unexpected sources. For example, a worker may realize that they are extremely frightened by the location of the crisis: this may be a drab, run-down tenement block; or they may be extremely inhibited by the presence of numerous individuals in the crisis situation, or by a claustrophobic atmosphere in a tiny room, or by the nature of the crisis itself – child abuse, marital strife, and so on. They must know why such challenges arise, and most important of all, they must be aware of natural tendencies to avoid such challenges. (See O'Hagan 1986 for conceptual frameworks enabling workers to explore their own vulnerabilities to these common features of crisis situations.) More seriously, the challenges may lie in certain discriminatory attitudes of the worker, similar, for example, to those sexist attitudes manifest in the behaviour of the police officers. The point made in the section on ethics, about opposing discrimination in all its forms, assumes added significance here.

4 Skills and techniques

All phases of crisis intervention contain difficulties and challenges. Surmounting these necessitates a repertoire of skills and techniques, many of which are standard tools in assessment, counselling, family therapy, and casework. 'Knowing' about the skills and techniques is insufficient of itself; there has to be abundant training, practice, and supervision in their application, specifically in and for crisis work. (The latter point is important: 'listening' and 'empathizing' in many crisis situations, for example, can be very different and much more challenging than listening to and empathizing with an individual client who is not in crisis.)

SUMMARY

This chapter began with examples of typical crisis situations which may at some point come to the attention of social workers. The purpose was to give some indication of the infinite number of crisis situations which can arise. It was immediately obvious that many of the cases had core gender, race, and structural components. The diversity of crisis situations makes it easy to understand the difficulty crisis pioneers had in attempting to find a suitable and lasting definition of crisis. A number of these attempts were explored, and the importance of the subjective experience in defining crisis was acknowledged. A brief survey of the literature and development of crisis intervention was provided, indicating a parallel diversity in theoretical orientations and practice models. The lasting benefits of the pioneers' work were acknowledged, but their lack of awareness about issues like race, gender, structural oppression, and discrimination, and how such issues impinge adversely upon the genesis and sustaining of crises processes had to be addressed.

Social work has made an invaluable contribution towards enhancing awareness about such issues. Crisis intervention is one of the most necessary and commonly applied methods of social work. Social work therefore has much to offer in securing the new foundations for an effective, modern crisis intervention service.

REFERENCES

Aguilera, D. C. and Messick, J. N. (1980) *Crisis Intervention: Theory and Methodology*, St. Louis: Mosby.

Bott, E. (1976) 'Hospital and society', *British Journal of Medical Society* 49: 97–140.

Caplan, G. (1961) *A Community Approach to Mental Health*, London: Tavistock.

Caplan, G. (1964) *Principles of Preventive Psychiatry*, New York: Basic Books.

Currer, C. (1991) 'Understanding the mother's viewpoint: the case of Pathan women in Britain', in S. Wyke and J. Hewison (eds) *Child Health Matters*, Milton Keynes: Open University Press.

Davis, A. (1991) 'A structural approach to social work', in *Social Work*, London: Jessica Kingsley, pp. 64–74.

Dominelli, L. (1988) *Anti-Racist Social Work*, London: Macmillan.

Eisler, R. M. and Hersen, N. (1973) 'Behavioural techniques in family oriented crisis intervention', *Archives of General Psychiatry* 28: 111–16.

Erikson, E. (1965) *Childhood and Society*, Harmondsworth: Penguin.

Langsley, D. G., Kaplan, D., Pittman, F. S., Machotka, P., Flomenhaft, K. and De Young, C. (1968) *The Treatment of Families in Crisis*, New York: Grune and Stratton.

Langsley, D. G., Machotka, P. and Flomenhaft, K. (1971) 'Avoiding mental hospital admission: a follow up study', *American Journal of Psychiatry*, 127 (10), pp. 1391–4.

Lindemann, E. (1944) 'Symptomatology and management of acute grief', *American Journal of Psychiatry* 101, reprinted in H. J. Parad (ed.) *Crisis Intervention, Selected Readings*, New York: Family Welfare Association, pp. 7–21.

O'Hagan, K. P. (1984) 'Family crisis intervention in social services', *Journal of Family Therapy* 6: 149–81.

O'Hagan, K. P. (1986) *Crisis Intervention in Social Services*, London: Macmillan.

O'Hagan, K. P. (1989) *Working with Child Sexual Abuse: A Post Cleveland Guide to Effective Principles and Practice*, Milton Keynes: Open University Press.

O'Hagan, K. P. (1991) 'Crisis intervention in social work', in J. Lishman (ed.) *Handbook of Theory for Practice Teachers in Social Work*, London: Jessica Kingsley, pp. 138–56.

O'Hagan, K. P. (1992) *The Emotional and Psychological Abuse of Children*, Buckingham: Open University Press.

Parad, H. K. and Caplan, G. (1965) 'A framework for studying families in crisis', in J. Parad (ed.) *Crisis Intervention: Selected Readings*, New York: Family Service Association of America, pp. 63–72.

Pittman, F. S. (1973) 'Managing acute psychiatric emergencies: defining the family crisis', in D. A. Bloch (ed.) *Techniques of Family Psychotherapy*, New York: Grune and Stratton.

Popay, J. (1991), 'Women, child care and money', in S. Wykes and J. Hewison, (eds) *Child Health Matters*, Milton Keynes: Open University Press.

Rapoport, L. (1971) 'Crisis intervention as a mode of brief treatment', in R. W.

Roberts and R. H. Nee (eds) *Comparative Theories in Social Casework*, Chicago: University of Chicago Press, pp. 267–311. Reprinted with minor changes in S. N. Katz (ed.) *Creativity in Social Work: Selected Writings of Lydia Rapoport*, Philadelphia: Temple University Press, pp. 83–124.

Scott, D. (1974) 'Cultural frontiers in the mental health service', *Schizophrenia Bulletin*, p.10.

Thompson, N. (1991) *Crisis Intervention Revisited*, Birmingham: Pepar.

Wright, B. (1991) *Sudden Death: Intervention Skills for the Caring Professionals*, London: Churchill Livingstone.

11 Casework

Celia Doyle

One of the most succinct yet accurate definitions of casework comes not from the plethora of textbooks with 'casework' in their title but from the *Oxford Illustrated Dictionary*. It defines casework as 'social work done by personal study of cases (individuals or families)'. This definition captures some of the essential features of casework: it is an approach used by social workers rather than other helping professionals; it involves 'study', the application of theories drawn from a range of social sciences to practice; it is a personal service and one which is offered to individuals or small groups of individuals in their family context.

'Casework' was once almost synonymous with the term 'social work'. However this is no longer true. There are many social workers who do not use a casework approach. The word is, in fact, no longer used so frequently in modern social work. It has however a long and, many would argue, honourable history.

HISTORICAL PERSPECTIVES

The origins of casework can be traced back to the latter part of the nineteenth century. The earliest known reference to 'caseworker' is to be found in the Proceedings of the National Conference in 1887 (Briar and Miller 1971: 4).

Social welfare provision in the nineteenth century was largely the responsibility of those charged with the task of administering the Poor Law, supplemented by a variety of charitable and philanthropic enterprises. In Britain in 1869 the Charity Organisation Society (COS) was formed, with a similar body being founded in America. The early representatives of the COS, the 'friendly visitors', were charged with the task of distinguishing between the 'deserving' and 'undeserving' poor. Friendly visitors had to determine on an individual or family basis which people were worthy of help. They could only do so by a thorough assessment. This meant that detailed records had to be kept and volunteer visitors had to be trained in how to make an assessment and record the information gathered.

At the same time, social reformers such as Robert Owen, Elizabeth Fry, Mary Carpenter and William Watson recognized that many of the problems of society lay not in the 'unworthy' individual but within society itself (Seed 1973: 18). Octavia Hill, another notable reformer, was concerned with environmental improvements in housing, supported the settlement movement founded by Samuel Barnett and was also actively involved with the COS. With her own deep respect for each individual, she was influential in changing attitudes towards those in need.

These developments meant that, by the early part of the twentieth century, casework in its modern form had emerged. The fact-finding assessment process was now so complicated that it could only be undertaken by trained professionals. Mary Richmond (1917), one of the pioneers of casework, defined it in her *Social Diagnosis* as a scientific and logical approach to social investigation (Briar and Miller 1971: 7). All individuals had an intrinsic worth and dignity and therefore deserved respect. The caseworker's job was not to determine who was deserving, but to assess how best an individual or a family could be helped and then to formulate and implement an appropriate treatment plan. Social, environmental, economic, personal and family factors were all to be taken into account. Furthermore the assessment could only be effectively made within the context of a friendly relationship between helper and helped.

The First World War saw the demise of the concept of deserving and undeserving as families and individuals from all walks of life, including the middle classes, required assistance and support. During and immediately after the war, the medical profession came to the fore of national consciousness. Not only were broken bodies healed by doctors but it seemed that broken minds, people suffering from shell shock, could be healed by psychiatrists. The work of Sigmund Freud appeared to give answers to so many mental and emotional problems. Caseworkers, seeking to increase their professionalism and the scientific basis of their work, embraced much that the medical profession, and psychiatry in particular, had to offer. In 1918 the Smith College in America opened one of the first training schools for psychiatric social workers.

This new psychiatric framework meant that if environmental and social factors could not supply a solution then the individual's inner world might be able to do so. However the Depression of the 1920s and 1930s meant that the environment again impinged. Lengthy in-depth psychoanalysis was seen as something of a luxury. A second Freud, Anna, in her *Ego and Mechanisms of Defense* published in 1946 offered a timely new framework from which emerged the Functional school. Its proponents believe that the ego, the conscious part of the individual, has its strengths and defences. People need not be the pawns of either environmental or internal unconscious forces

(Gambrill 1983). Instead, the caseworker's task is to help clients to discover and release their own coping mechanisms. Client motivation and co-operation were key concepts.

The Second World War saw the culmination of the suffering which had started with the Depression. In the ensuing peace there were hopes of a brave new world in which poverty and suffering on the scale seen before and during the wars would be obliterated. Britain saw the emergence of the welfare state in which both medical and social work professions were to make a significant contribution. However, as the state played an increasing part in welfare provision, its agents had to act in a social control role. As concern about delinquency and 'problem families' grew in the 1950s social workers found themselves exercising authority and working with uncooperative clients. This necessitated the development of new casework models.

By the late 1950s Helen Perlman was offering the world of social work her problem-solving framework. She criticized the study–diagnosis–treatment model of earlier workers for producing 'more problem-solving activity on the caseworker's part than on the client's' (Perlman 1957: 61). She therefore advocated improving the client's own problem-solving capacities.

The 1960s saw the development of the Diagnostic or Psychosocial school, which again has much in common with the Functional school. One of its greatest proponents was Florence Hollis. She identified four major casework processes: environmental modification; psychological support; clarification or increasing the client's ability to see external realities clearly; and insight-giving to enable the client to understand the influence of past and current emotions. She also acknowledged that 'there is such a thing as professional authority... and under certain circumstances it can be put to very good use' (Hollis 1964: 97).

The Psychosocial school emphasizes assessment and the casework relationship. It seeks to rectify problems in the environment, while enhancing the client's own ego strengths or coping mechanisms by support and clarification. But, in its endorsement of insight-giving, it draws on psychodynamic therapies.

Although the Psychosocial school had a considerable influence on social work, it was not without its critics. Firstly, psychoanalysis and insight-giving all required relatively prolonged intervention. Some clients could not afford to wait. Furthermore as William Reid and Ann Shyne, the exponents of 'brief casework' explain, 'While caseworkers continue to be in short supply, the clienteles of casework continue to grow' (1969: 1). This meant that there was a search for faster and more economical treatment methods. There emerged not only 'brief' as opposed to 'extended' casework but also 'task-centred casework' (Reid and Epstein 1972). The latter typically involves about twelve sessions. The caseworker and client agree tasks and objectives which are then worked on by the client between treatment sessions.

Secondly, it became obvious that prolonged assessment, insight-giving and support did not always elicit any real change. There was also concern that psychosocial methods were only effective with certain groups, particularly those who were fairly articulate and could respond to verbal reasoning. By the early 1960s, clinical psychologists had started using behaviour modification to good effect. This offered an efficient, economical method of intervention which was seen to be effective with a wide range of hitherto intractable problems (Jehu *et al.* 1972; Schwartz *et al.* 1975; Fischer 1978). Behavioural casework became a popular method of intervention.

As earlier theories were challenged and fresh ideas were gathered from the social sciences, new models blossomed until, by the 1980s, there was an almost overwhelming number of theoretical frameworks for caseworkers to choose from. To those already mentioned could be added: cognitive therapies (Fischer 1978); crisis intervention (Rapoport 1970); family therapy; competency-based casework (Gambrill 1983); Gestalt therapy; transactional analysis (Berne 1961); a systems approach; role theory models. Jeff Hopkins, in 1986, was able to itemize twenty-six different models on which caseworkers could base their intervention.

All these divergent frameworks and models are nevertheless united by a set of core values and an emphasis on the casework relationship. It is these unifying principles which will be examined in the following sections of this chapter. However, before continuing the theoretical discussion a particular piece of intervention, illustrating the efficacy of casework, will be described.

CASE STUDY – THE 'S' FAMILY

This case study recalls real events. The family members at the centre of this study have given their permission for their story to be used to inform and educate other helping professionals. However all identifying details have been changed. First names are used when referring to family members because this was their own stated preference.

Tom, at the age of 30, was left with three young children after his wife had found a new partner. A skilled but poorly paid worker, he nevertheless wanted to keep his job, so he advertised for a housekeeper. Pam, aged 17 years old, was appointed. Pam's own family lived nearby. Her mother had alcohol problems. Under the influence of drink, she could be violent towards her three children, Pam, Jane and Joe. Pam had no contact with her father who had disappeared shortly after Joe's birth.

After a couple of years Pam and Tom married. Tom's three children had always been rather antagonistic to Pam. Their relationship with their stepmother deteriorated further when she gave birth to a baby son, Dan. A number of weeks later Tom was rushed to hospital with a serious heart condition. He was not expected to survive.

Days later Pam's younger brother and sister arrived asking for protection because their mother was drinking heavily and physically abusing them. They moved in. Their mother responded by regularly coming to Pam's house at night, creating a commotion outside. The neighbours were soon complaining about the noise.

Social services responded by taking the three step-children into voluntary, short-term care as Pam was becoming increasingly depressed and exhausted. Dan was by now fretful and demanding.

Tom began to recover and, although needing intensive nursing care, was discharged home. His illness had left him with sight and hearing impairments. The social services at this point determined that the three step-children could return home.

Pam, now barely 20, was faced with the prospect of caring for six children including a young baby and a very sick husband, on slim finances in a two-bedroomed house. She had no real support. Her mother was still causing commotions day and night and the neighbours were hostile. One night Pam, feeling desperately tired and depressed, could not cope with Dan's crying. She wanted him to be quiet and let her get some sleep. She held his neck too tightly and the child died.

Pam was charged with unlawful killing and was placed on probation. She received psychiatric help for her depression. The three step-children remained in care but visited regularly. Joe and Jane returned to their mother who sought help for her drink problem. Tom despite his very many losses remained a source of strength and support for his wife.

Two years later Pam again became pregnant. Both she and Tom wanted to keep the baby and were willing to accept any monitoring and support that the authorities felt was necessary. It was agreed that they should do so with voluntary supervision. By the time of the baby's birth the Probation Order had virtually come to an end. Therefore, the family was allocated a specialist caseworker.

Although, ever since the death of Dan, the family had been carefully assessed, one of the first tasks of the caseworker was to evaluate the strengths and vulnerabilities of the family. Problems which might create undue stress were identified and ways found of coping with each problem as it arose.

The caseworker used a variety of ways of alleviating problems. Sometimes material assistance was appropriate. Verbal therapies were employed when helping Tom recognize and express his anger about his losses or when acknowledging with Pam her very real abilities as a mother. The caseworker used local contacts to mobilize the community into supporting rather than condemning the parents. She also drew on the expertise of other professionals, such as a specialist social worker for the hearing impaired, when Tom's deteriorating hearing demanded new ways of communication.

The 'S' family required a lot of help and reassurance until the new baby, Ross, reached the age at which Dan died. When he survived the first nine months the parents' confidence grew. When he was a year old the caseworker's visits and support diminished. Just after his second birthday the caseworker, with the agreement and understanding of the family, withdrew from formal contact. A few years later she learnt that Ross was making good progress and he now had a younger brother. The family had not needed the assistance of the social services since Ross was a toddler.

The parents expressed the view that without the caseworker's help, even had Ross survived babyhood unharmed, they would have had a very hard physical and emotional struggle. Instead they derived great joy from his early months and years. The caseworker gave practical assistance but also helped Pam and Tom mobilize their own strengths. It is debatable whether any other form of intervention would have met the family's many needs in so comprehensive a fashion.

THE CASEWORK RELATIONSHIP

The Charity Organisation Societies in America and Britain were concerned that the discharge of charitable welfare services should be placed on a scientific basis. This meant that a thorough, methodical assessment had to take place. But in order to do so the friendly visitors, the forerunners of caseworkers, had to form a positive relationship with the people they were trying to help.

The primary importance of the relationship became one of the distinguishing features of casework. Elements of the casework relationship have evolved and changed but its core has remained much the same since the earlier part of the twentieth century. It does not have the mutuality of a friend–friend relationship, nor the deep, penetrating, emotional components of the parent–child or psychoanalyst–patient relationship. By the 1960s, Felix Biestek (1961: 12) was able to define it as 'The dynamic interaction of attitudes and emotions between the caseworker and the client, with the purpose of helping the client achieve a better adjustment between himself and his environment'.

Identifying the client

A 'case' can be an individual client or a group of clients in a family situation. One problem encountered by many social workers, especially those working with families, is the identification of the client: the person with whom they form a relationship and on whose behalf they act.

In the case of the 'S' family Tom, Pam and Ross were all 'clients'. The caseworker was able to form a relationship with each family member because the over-riding objective, that of ensuring that Ross was not harmed, was the same for each family member. The family was not in conflict. Assistance given directly to one member was indirect assistance to the other two. For example, provision of counselling for Tom helped him to cope with his losses, but it also benefited Pam and Ross because it gave Tom the emotional space and strength to meet their need for his affection and support.

However, problems arise for social workers attempting casework with couples, groups or families when the wishes of some members are in direct conflict with the wishes and interests of other members. Nothing has thrown this into greater relief in recent years than cases of child sexual abuse within the family. An illustration of this is the case of the 'B' family. Its members have again given permission for their story to be told although, as always, identifying details have been changed.

One night, Mr B attempted to rape Ruth, his 12–year-old daughter. Mr B claimed that he had been drunk, had climbed into the wrong bed and had started to have intercourse with the person he thought was his wife.

There had been a history of conflict between Ruth and her father, caused possibly by Mr B's attempts to 'groom' his daughter by a combination of intimidation and seduction before attempting to rape her. The assault was, as far as Ruth was concerned, the 'last straw'. She could no longer trust her father and she did not want to live with him in the same household.

Mr B moved out temporarily but wished to return home. He had convinced himself that he had made an innocent mistake. He was very fond not only of his wife and Ruth but also of his 6–year-old daughter, Dora.

Mrs B found that when her husband left the household she was struggling to cope without his support. She was lonely and hoped for his return. She felt angry with Ruth, although she was not sure why, but did not want her to leave. She was also worried in case her husband attempted to assault Dora.

Dora, for her part, longed to have her father back home again. She did not understand what had happened and was angry with Ruth for 'causing a fuss'.

There was a maelstrom of intense emotions and conflicts within the family. The sexual assault had not only brought these out in the open but had intensified them. Any single caseworker trying to meet the varying demands and needs of each family member was doomed to fail. One of the reasons why traditional casework fell into disfavour in the late 1980s was because attempts by lone caseworkers to intervene in this type of family situation were totally ineffective. Lone workers tended to become sucked into the family system, becoming overpowered by the most powerful family member, who was usually the abuser. They then colluded against the victim and vulnerable family members or, alternatively, identified too closely with the victim and became overwhelmed by feelings of helplessness and hopelessness.

This danger was avoided in the case of the 'B' family because three caseworkers were involved. One social worker was charged with the task of helping Ruth and a second helped Mrs B and Dora. Mr B admitted the sexual assault, although denied attempted rape, and was put on probation. He was therefore allocated a probation officer. Each caseworker was able to form a positive relationship with their particular family member and each knew who their client was. In order to prevent destructive family conflicts being mirrored by the team of caseworkers, a case co-ordinator was appointed to identify and facilitate constructive coping strategies.

Underpinning principles

Central to casework is the concept of respect for each and every person. This respect transcends a person's role, status or behaviour. Some people may be admired more than others because they have special skills or attributes, but caseworkers afford all individuals, whatever their personal qualities, equal respect. The poor, the weak, the ill educated, the social outcast is given the same high regard as the wealthy, the strong, the highly educated or the socially acclaimed.

The dictionary includes in its definitions of the verb to respect 'to treat with consideration'. This is an essential feature for all caseworkers. Furthermore, they treat each and every client with the same degree of consideration. Caseworkers do not discriminate on grounds of colour, class, race or religion, an important value in our multiracial society. Nor do they discriminate on grounds of gender, age or disability. They do however take these factors into account when assessing the best method of responding to need.

Raymond Plant (1970) argues that the core concept in casework is that of respect for persons. He claims that other concepts or principles, such as 'individualization' or 'self-determination', are 'merely elucidations of various emphases within that concept' (Plant 1970: 9). A number of principles, supporting and expanding on respect for persons, have been identified by theorists.

Felix Biestek (1961) discussed seven principles of the casework relationship. These are individualization, confidentiality, acceptance, non-judgemental attitudes, controlled emotional involvement, purposeful expression of feelings, and lastly, client self-determination.

Individualization

Under the Poor Law all people in need were seen as a burden to be disposed of as efficiently as possible. Little account was taken of individual circumstances. Paupers formed a homogeneous group or at best two groups, the 'worthy' and the 'unworthy'. As mentioned, pioneers from Elizabeth Fry to Mary Richmond changed this attitude. They embraced the view that human beings are united in that they all have a basic worth and dignity but all are separated by each person's own unique qualities and situations.

Caseworkers therefore will as far as possible avoid stereotypes and labels. While they will recognize that, for example, all women or all black people share a common history of discrimination, they will also be aware that each individual woman or black person will have his or her own unique experience and perception of discrimination.

Confidentiality

As Biestek so aptly explains, when a person comes seeking assistance from a social work agency 'he definitely does not want to exchange his reputation for the casework help he is seeking' (Biestek 1961: 121). Caseworkers will keep to themselves private information about clients, unless they have to share it with others in order to gain appropriate help for their client and, sometimes, to ensure the safety of other people.

The ground rules to sharing information are: that the client should be told what is to be shared, when, how and why; that disclosure is restricted to those people who have to be told; that only essential information is shared.

Acceptance

This is the ability of the caseworker to maintain respect for clients despite their negative attributes and behaviour. It is tolerant understanding and acknowledgement of the reality of the client's feelings even if the caseworker cannot truly share them. Carl Rogers' term 'unconditional positive regard' summarizes the concept of acceptance (Pippin 1980: 27).

Acceptance is 'conveyed by the worker's interest and concern, and by the constancy of that response despite negative response or deviant behaviour on the part of the client' (Davison 1965: 17). It is demonstrated by warmth and empathy on the part of the caseworker. Empathy is the ability to understand another person's world and to communicate that understanding by active listening and responding (Fischer 1978: 192).

Non-judgemental attitudes

Caseworkers are not concerned with evaluating the moral worth of a client. It is however 'legitimate to assess and evaluate his qualities and potential' (Foren and Bailey 1968: 38). In practical terms this means that social workers, for example working with child sex abusers, will refrain from imposing moralistic labels on their clients. However, they will challenge the abusers' attempts to minimize, rationalize and excuse their abusive behaviour. They will also legitimately probe the abusers' attitudes and belief systems in order to evaluate how far they pose a risk to vulnerable children.

Effective communication of feeling

Moffett (1968) usefully links two of Biestek's principles – 'purposeful expression of feeling' and 'controlled emotional involvement' together under this heading. Purposeful expression of feeling relates to non-judgemental attitudes, in that clients have the right to talk about and show their feelings, including negative feelings, without being condemned by the caseworker. Instead the worker will be sensitive to the client's feelings, try to understand and give a 'purposeful, appropriate response' (Biestek 1961: 50).

Client self-determination

This is not the same as encouraging clients to do exactly what they want whatever the circumstances. It means respecting clients' wishes, rights, capacity for self-knowledge and responsibility for their own actions. It is an expedience as well as a principle, because in practical terms people resist being told what to do. Externally imposed change is usually only temporary; permanent change comes from within.

There are occasions when caseworkers will make use of authority invested in them by virtue of their role or by law. This is sometimes necessary because clients are not always governed by conscious decisions or by awareness of the consequences of their actions. 'The client left to follow impulse, or driven by it, is not self-determining' (Parker 1972: 21).

THE FUTURE FOR CASEWORK

The last two decades of the twentieth century have seen a revolution in social work. It has been forced to adopt and adapt the language and concepts of the market place. 'Casework', as a term, has given way to 'case management'. Social work agencies are care 'providers' and 'purchasers'. Clients are 'users', 'customers' or 'consumers'. Once social work borrowed from the medical profession with the use of terms such as 'patient', 'diagnosis' and 'treatment'. For a brief period it seemed to find its own terminology with 'client', 'assessment', 'intervention' and 'casework'. Now it has lost this identity and is borrowing and embracing the terminology and concepts of the world of business.

Casework processes are not, in fact, that far removed from general managerial models. Good management starts with the identification of needs and an understanding of the values and principles underpinning any response to these needs. This is much the same process propounded by social casework theorists, hence the very many textbooks devoted to a discussion of the values and principles of casework.

Effective managers then define the purpose of any action and identify goals, aims and objectives. This is also the task of the effective social caseworker.

Setting priorities, devising strategies and formulating plans form the next stage of both the management process and the casework process. For some social work interventions, such as task-centred casework, prioritizing goals and objectives is of paramount importance.

The action stage follows, as both manager and caseworker co-ordinate and implement plans. For managers, this might be to engage in a team-building exercise with his or her staff group. For the caseworker, action might be to obtain a material resource or to provide bereavement counselling. In both instances the action will only be effective if there has been early planning and preparation and if the staff group or client have been actively engaged in the process. Neither manager nor caseworker can act in isolation.

The final stage is that of monitoring, review and evaluation. In the past caseworkers, especially those from the psychodynamic schools, have perhaps paid too little attention to monitoring and review, concentrating instead on how best to disengage from a client. However, this stage now has a higher profile in social work in general in the wake of a number of highly publicized tragedies and scandals and the attendant media interest.

Just as the friendly visitor of the nineteenth century evolved into the caseworker of the twentieth century, so present-day caseworkers may well enter the twenty-first century as case managers. Social work itself having drawn on the physical and medical sciences in the last century and having applied theory from the social sciences in this one, may well base intervention on the business and management sciences in the century to come.

It is to be hoped, however, that even if the terminology and theoretical frameworks change, most of the principles of casework are retained. If society loses sight of the value and uniqueness of each individual then the struggle against oppression and the abuse of power will be diminished. Jacqueline Spring, an incest survivor, wrote in her autobiography:

> When I read about concentration camps, I am drawn again and again to speculate on what made men and women able to live comfortably in the midst of such devastation without seeming to have any feelings for the suffering they were inflicting, or allowing to be inflicted, upon fellow human beings. The answer of course is, that it was only possible for them because they did not see the prisoners as fellow human beings.
>
> (1987: 51).

Social work must continue to demand what caseworkers throughout this century have demanded: that all people are respected, are accepted and have a right to confidentiality, to self-determination and to the expression of feelings. Only in this way will the de-personalization of vulnerable or minority groups be countered. Only by resisting the objectification of the members of such groups can society ensure they are protected from oppression. Only by valuing each individual may a return to the terms 'undeserving' and 'unworthy', applied to people in need, be avoided.

REFERENCES

Berne, E. (1961) *Transactional Analysis in Psychotherapy*, New York: Condor.

Biestek, F. P. (1961) *The Casework Relationship*, London: Allen & Unwin.

Briar, S. and Miller, H. (1971) *Problems and Issues in Social Casework*, New York: Columbia University Press.

Davison, E. H. (1965) *Social Casework: A Basic Textbook for Students of Casework and for Administrators in the Social Services*, 2nd edn 1970, London: Baillière, Tindall & Cassell.

Fischer, J. (1978) *Effective Casework Practice: An Eclectic Approach*, New York: McGraw-Hill.

Foren, R. and Bailey, R. (1968) *Authority in Social Casework*, Oxford: Pergamon Press.

Freud, A. (1946) *The Ego and the Mechanisms of Defense*, New York: International Universities Press.

Gambrill, E. (1983) *Casework: A Competency-Based Approach*, New Jersey: Prentice-Hall.

Hollis, F. (1964) *Casework: A Psychosocial Therapy*, 2nd edn 1972, New York: Random House.

Hopkins, J. (1986) *Caseworker: A Guide to the Informed and Sensitive Practice of Social Casework*, Birmingham: Pepar.

Jehu, D., Hardiker, P., Yelloly, M. and Stone, M. (1972) *Behaviour Modification in Social Work*, Chichester: Wiley.

Moffett, J. (1968) *Concepts in Casework Treatment*, London: Routledge & Kegan Paul.

Parker, G. (ed.) (1972) *Casework Within Social Work*, Newcastle: Department of Social Studies, University of Newcastle upon Tyne.

Perlman, H. H. (1957) *Social Casework: A Problem-solving Process*, Chicago: University of Chicago Press.

Pippin, J. A. (1980) *Developing Casework Skills*, Beverly Hills: Sage.

Plant, R. (1970) *Social and Moral Theory in Casework*, London: Routledge & Kegan Paul.

Rapoport, L. (1970) 'Crisis intervention as a mode of treatment' in R. W. Roberts and R. H. Nee (eds) *Theories of Social Casework*, Chicago: University of Chicago Press.

Reid, W. J. and Epstein, L. (1972) *Task Centred Casework*, New York: Columbia University Press.

Reid, W. J. and Shyne, A. W. (1969) *Brief and Extended Casework*, New York: Columbia University Press.

Richmond, M. E. (1917) *Social Diagnosis*, New York: Russel Sage Foundation.

Schwartz, A., Goldiamond, I. and Howe, M. W. (1975) *Social Casework: A Behavioural Approach*, New York: Columbia University Press.

Seed, P. (1973) *The Expansion of Social Work in Britain*, London: Routledge & Kegan Paul.

Spring, J. (1987) *Cry Hard and Swim: The Story of an Incest Survivor*, London: Virago.

FURTHER READING

Bamford, T. (1990) *The Future of Social Work*, London: Macmillan.

Roberts, R. W. and Nee, R. H. (eds) (1970) *Theories of Social Casework*, Chicago: University of Chicago Press.

Sainsbury, E. (1970) *Social Diagnosis in Casework*, London: Routledge & Kegan Paul.

Timms, N. (1968) *The Language of Social Casework*, London: Routledge & Kegan Paul.

Younghusband, E. (1966) *New Developments in Casework*, London: Allen & Unwin.

12 Family therapy

Philippa Seligman

Newly qualified as a social worker in 1972, I had been in my child guidance clinic job for a couple of weeks when I caught on to two very important beliefs which were firmly embedded in the system. One of the family therapy pioneers, Virginia Satir, used to say that the era of the immaculate conception still reigned supreme and so it occurred to no one that fathers might be invited to discuss their child's doings or misdoings, and the other belief was that Psychiatrists Rule OK and so, in the hierarchy of clinic teams, social workers were outdone in lowliness only by students, secretaries and cleaners – the two latter categories being all-female. Encouraged by a progressive family therapy lecturer on my course and emboldened by the award of my qualifying certificates, I challenged these beliefs in one memorable conversation with the psychiatrist prior to a session where the doctor would interview the child and, based on my report of a home visit, write a report of her own whilst I 'chatted to' the mother.

Why, I asked, could I not join the doctor and together we could talk to mother, child and father who was sitting in the car outside? The psychiatrist paled, clutched her desk to stop from falling off her chair and said in a faint voice that she thought that might be very risky. However, we did indeed try it as did many such teams in Britain in those years. The rest, as they say, is history.

And what an interesting history it is. An evolution of quite dramatic proportions which took the social work scene in this country from the grossly misinterpreted Seebohm Report (when his plea for generic teams turned into a panic to train generic workers and to look askance upon specialisms), through the hugely influential waves of new techniques from the USA – sensitivity groups, encounter groups, Gestalt therapy, transactional analysis and so on – to the gradual introduction of phrases such as conjoint family work, interactional framework and family therapy. Family therapy is an approach which adopts the stance that explanations and solutions to human problems lie in the understanding of past and current relationships between significantly linked people rather than within each individual. Since the family, in one form or another, is still the most powerfully influential system in western society, the approach is known as family therapy even though the whole family may not attend the therapy sessions. Individuals and couples are frequently seen on their own and, indeed, the method may also be applied to large organizational systems which seek consultation. However, the focus on context and process takes precedence over content. Patterns of behaviours and beliefs will be explored more than feelings and emotions and the overall emphasis will be upon creating opportunities for new patterns to evolve.

The textbooks were mostly American until, in the mid and late 1970s, that magical and often misunderstood word 'paradox' was tripping from everyone's lips. The Milan group of Mara Selvini Palazzoli, Juliana Prata, Luigi Boscolo and Gianfranco Cecchin wrote a book (Palazzoli *et al.* 1978) describing their work of the previous decade with 'families in schizophrenic transaction'. Translated into English by Cecchin's (then) wife Elizabeth Burt, the book seemed to strike a collective nerve in the social work world and in the wider field of the helping professions. Hot debates arose which, at their most polarized, accepted the work of the Milan group and, in particular, of the technique of paradoxical injunctions, as a therapeutic wondrous magic or else damned it as unethical hocus-pocus with evil intent. That neither view was accurate did not detract from the welcome spurt of creativity which occurred in Europe, including the UK, when for the first time we began to see textbooks and journal papers on family therapy from our own side of the Atlantic.

In 1976 the Association for Family Therapy was inaugurated and within two years some European, English and Welsh family therapists were being invited to present their work in the USA. The traffic was no longer one way! Family institutes and centres specializing in marital and family work became established and training courses in family therapy were set up and eagerly attended by increasing numbers of social workers. There was an almost missionary zeal which, when faced with scepticism and opposition on grounds of ethics, theoretical validity and economic resources only became stronger.

Perhaps inevitably, factions arose within the family therapy field itself and a number of different major schools emerged. Virginia Satir, a social worker herself, was the propounder of communications theory for family work and there was a distinct flavour of healing, rescuing and generally making-it-better which I believe appealed strongly to social workers. Salvador Minuchin, a psychiatrist at the Philadelphia Child Guidance Clinic, wrote of his work and founded the school of structural therapy, so called because the family was viewed as a system of structures based on hierarchies, role models and boundaries both within the family group and between it and the outside world. As in Satir's model, the therapist was active, directive and aiming at change to a more functional family interaction with fairly frequent sessions. In a small town in California the Mental Research Institute at Palo Alto was the main centre for Brief therapy where although primarily looking at relationships (as opposed to intra-psychic phenomena in individuals), therapists were problem focused and therapy ended when the presenting problem was resolved. Where others, at that time, insisted on seeing whole families, these Brief therapists preferred to work with only those members of the family actively wishing to come to sessions who were sometimes referred to as 'customers'. Writings by John Weakland, Richard Fish, Paul Watslawick and John Haley were, perhaps, the best known in the 1970s and 1980s although many other familiar names were involved in the evolution of Brief and Strategic therapies (see Barker 1986, chapter 1).

All of these approaches were taken up and practised in the UK to some extent. Structural therapy was, perhaps, the most popular and therefore, not surprisingly, the most threatened when 'Milan' or 'Milan-systemic' ideas seemed to sweep across Britain, Europe and even the USA. There were similarities but these were largely overlooked, so great were the differences in concept and in practice between these two. Like the old nursery rhyme of the lion and the unicorn who fought for the crown, the field split like boxing promoters wanting to pit Minuchin against the Milan group and, indeed, some pitched battles (called study days or two-day conferences!) were set up almost as gladiatorial contests. The combatants, however, refused to fight and the audiences were left to continue their own arguments. Although both schools claimed to view the family as a system and drew upon general systems theory, the Milan team had extended the concepts to include the therapist and the (by now established) therapeutic team in their thinking and the differences were becoming more apparent. The two men in the Milan team had separated from the two women (all four of them are psychiatrists) and the women had set up a new centre mainly concentrating on research. Where structural therapy aimed to 'join with' or 'engage' the family and then confront, challenge, re-arrange, support, manipulate and change the family to a more healthy functioning, the Milan therapy stressed therapeutic neutrality, information gathering by means of circular questioning, a stance of non-blaming, non-pathologizing and, most startling, an apparent indifference to change (the inherent paradox) and a positive disinterest in precisely *how* the family changed if, indeed, it chose to do so. Therapy was brief – six to ten sessions – where structuralists might work over twenty sessions. Some structural therapists combined with brief therapy and offered 'contracts' of up to six sessions where the Milan followers regarded each session as a new consultation working on the fresh information gained by the response to the previous session's intervention and the 'news of difference' from the longish interval between sessions, usually one month compared with the weekly or fortnightly structuralists. Structuralists provoked and rehearsed families to change within sessions, often re-arranging seating, staging role reversals and dialogues between family members, supporting them through these ventures and working closely with them. Milan disciples adopted the position of the 'curious observer', less concerned about overt expressions of empathy in the belief that stimulating people's curiosity about their own relationship patterns would enable them to make choices about changes which they saw as desirable (that is, rather than those which the therapist saw as desirable).

During the 1980s, many more centres for training in family therapy became established and the bulk of those taking Diploma and MSc courses are social workers. Courses may be recognized by the Central Council for Education and Training in Social Work, validated by universities and registered by the Association for Family Therapy so that these qualifications have become both sought after and increasingly accepted in social work agencies. In the UK some posts carry a family therapy title and some people describe themselves as family therapists, but the majority of professionals using family therapy as an approach may describe themselves as social workers, psychologists, psychiatrists, community psychiatric nurses and so on.[1]

While some family therapists become known for working with a particular client group – for example, bereavement and illness, divorce and separation, life stages (the very young or the elderly), step-families, or with specific problems such as substance abuse, school non-attendance, AIDS/HIV – more usually the systemic framework frees workers to work therapeutically and effectively with a wide range of problems, with a variety of client groups.

A few case examples will illustrate this.

Mrs Allen and Katie (I have used pseudonyms to protect confidentiality) had been receiving help from their social services department for some ten years. There has been a violent marriage, a bitter and stressful divorce and an abundance of problems concerning housing, money and the well-being of the four children. Katie, aged 8, was the youngest – she was 3 years old when Mrs Allen finally succeeded in obtaining a divorce. Their social worker, the latest in a long line, had sought family therapy because of a recent event and its aftermath. About a year before, Katie was in the house of a neighbour and she was sexually abused by the man in the house. The man had been convicted and imprisoned but was about to be released. Katie had suffered from nightmares for years especially following violent episodes between her parents and these had become worse in intensity and frequency since the assault upon her. Recently, knowing her attacker was due to return to the neighbourhood, Katie had run into the house screaming hysterically saying that she had seen Des (the man). Mrs Allen, telling me this story, said in order to calm the child, she had slapped her across the face a couple of times. Katie sat huddled at the back of the interview room looking forlorn and miserable and Mrs Allen said doubtfully 'Well, I'm sorry, love, but it was the only thing I could do, wasn't it?'.

My initial feeling of shock at the situation where a terrified and abused child rushes to mother only to receive a slap, gave way to a more neutral view of a woman, herself abused, struggling to do her best with Katie, frightened and guilty over the attack on her daughter by a man thought to be a harmless neighbour and lacking confidence in her own parenting skills. She had, in some ways, received so much help and support from social workers that she relied almost totally on them to show her what to do and, to their credit, they had never let her down. However, she could not visualize her life without a social worker as part of her family system.

I began exploring the relationship between Katie and her mother. That they loved each other was beyond doubt but it seemed that, as a result of seeing her mother as a 'victim', Katie had become the protective one and Mrs Allen, the helpless and dependent one in the relationship. When Katie dramatically needed her mother's help, things went out of control and Mrs Allen panicked. She had also held the notion that Katie somehow blamed her for the failure of the marriage and the violent behaviour of her husband against whom the child had tried to protect her. On that basis, she saw any naughty or disturbed behaviour on Katie's part as directed against herself.

We worked together to increase Mrs Allen's skills and resources in parenting and to increase her confidence in her own competence. After a few sessions, her social worker was successful in obtaining a house for the family in another area where they would not see Des. She was delighted and saw only one snag – that this would mean a change of social worker and she got on so well with the current worker. I risked some humour, in the light of the marked changes and progress I had observed. 'Oh, Mrs Allen,' I teased, 'I have this picture of you on your 70th birthday [she was only 38!] with a cake and all the candles – and you sending for a social worker to help blow them out!' She laughed and then became thoughtful. Then she made a decision. She would allow herself to be 'allocated' so that she had a name to call in case of need but she would ask them to wait and see if she needed help. 'I'll see how far we go for a few months', she said. In fact, Mrs Allen had done a really good job of supporting Katie and the nightmares were only occasional now. When I asked Katie when she thought her mother would stop being upset about Des she replied 'Never'. 'And what about you? When will you stop being upset?' She considered carefully and then smiled and said 'When I am 9'. She was 8 years and 8 months old at the time.

In another case, a distraught woman asked for an appointment saying 'something terrible had happened' with her 14-year-old daughter. She agreed to invite her husband and daughter to the session but declined to bring a younger son. The family lived in a small suburban community on the outskirts of a city and all the residents knew each other well – their children went to school together.

Mr and Mrs Harris arrived looking agitated and sat on either side of Sarah. There was some embarrassed negotiation about who would start to tell me why they had come. Sarah shook her head and indicated that her mother should speak and then became more and more sulky-looking as the story unfolded. The Harrises had received a 'phone call late one evening about a week ago when they believed Sarah to be at a girlfriend's house. The call was from the parents of a boy in the neighbourhood saying that the Harrises should go and collect Sarah because there had been some kind of trouble. It turned out that, upon returning home, the boy's parents had discovered their son with four or five other boys of 16 and 17 in a bedroom with Sarah. The boys were reasonably clothed while Sarah was naked. Some alcohol had been drunk and, naturally, an almighty row had ensued when they were discovered.

In the wake of this incident, Sarah had been grounded for one month but the atmosphere in the family was angry and tense with Sarah becoming increasingly truculent and bad-tempered, Mr Harris furious and threatening whilst Mrs Harris veered between distress, tearfulness and shocked anger. They could barely have a conversation with their daughter and talked about her rather than to her for the first fifteen minutes of the session. The parents of one of the boys involved had contacted the social services department and were awaiting a visit from a social worker but the Harrises felt that this was too drastic a step for them and had come to me in the hope that this could be avoided.

Sarah's account of the events of the evening was that three of the boys had been known to her and had invited her and another girl to the house to talk, play music, drink coffee and sit around together 'for a laugh'. She had not had any alcohol but when the boys suggested playing strip poker she had risen to the challenge and agreed. The other girl said she had to be home early and had left at about 10.30 pm when things were becoming 'a bit funny'.

Mr and Mrs Harris, clearly wanting to believe the story but also too upset and worried to accept Sarah's account, looked helpless, frowning and sighing. Sarah, struggling to retain some dignity and semblance of credibility, adopted a stance of 'toughing it out'. She was, despite the scowling looks she gave her parents, an attractive girl trying hard to seem older than her years and the way she spoke indicated that she generally gave her parents plenty of reason to trust her to act responsibly even though she was often rebellious and argumentative, too. By the time we were about half-way through our first session, all three were calmer and more interested in answering my questions. I was beginning to build a sense of how Sarah, her brother, her mother and father related to each other and what their beliefs were on a range of topics such as child-rearing, gender roles, dependence and independence and the ways in which emotions were dealt with in this family.

My sense was of a united and caring family frightened and angry over what the parents saw as an unacceptable level of dangerously rebellious and foolish behaviour by their daughter and which Sarah was determined to brazen out in the face of what she experienced as intolerably heavy-handed and rigid attitudes by her 'old-fashioned' parents. My usual way of interviewing is to explore the context thoroughly to gain a broad understanding of the clients' background, beliefs, resources and so on. In this case, my move to encompass the wider family relationships proved a turning point. As I sought information about Mr and Mrs Harris's families of origin, I learned that Mr Harris's mother had died a year ago. He gave the information calmly and with no trace of distress and I turned to Sarah to say 'Was this grandma special to you? Were you close?'. The girl nodded, flushed deeply and began to weep copiously. Her parents glanced at each other in surprise and then at her with concern. 'Are you surprised at Sarah's response?' I asked. They had known she was upset but not that she still felt so strongly about her gran's death. Mr Harris's eyes were moist. Mrs Harris passed Sarah a tissue and touched her shoulder comfortingly. This was not a time to ask more questions but a significant moment and one which could be used positively. Sarah, tears flowing, nodded when I said to her 'You are still very sad and miss your gran a lot'. I turned to her parents, 'I think Sarah's telling you something really important right now.' The atmosphere was tense and emotional as I went on, 'She has learned well all that you are teaching her about growing up. She often shows how independent and creative she can be. She tests herself as an emerging young woman, tests her ideas by arguing with you and sometimes, of course, she goes too far. So she is also showing you now that part of her still feels like the vulnerable little girl who can get out of her depth and be scared of being out of control. She's telling you that part of her still needs your love and your guidance as she continues to 'grow up'.' I paused noting that they were all very attentive and nodding at my comments.

Sarah dried her eyes, blew her nose – and grinned. 'It did happen exactly as I told you', she said. 'Honestly, nothing else happened – I wouldn't have let it go any further. I wished I'd got out sooner but I just didn't know how to without looking silly. And I ended up making a fool of myself anyway. It was so embarrassing.' She had become serious and her parents responded by reassuring her both of their love and of the fact that she was still grounded for a month!

The session ended with the feeling that at least they would now be able to talk to each other. They requested one more session to discuss more general and indeed more usual parent–teenager frustration and by the end of the second session, they felt able to face the future again.

Another case is that of a young man of 19 referred by his general practitioner for drug abuse and 'paranoid behaviour'. Mr and Mrs Phillips and another son, Gordon, aged 17, agreed to come with Mike to the first session. Mike was very withdrawn and inarticulate but maintained that he had only tried 'acid' a few times a couple of months ago and had now even stopped smoking cannabis which, in any case, he did not consider harmful. His parents, on the other hand, were extremely alarmed at the thought of drugs but accepted that it was natural to drink moderately. While Mike had been average at school and was said to be quite artistic, he had never had a good job and had been unemployed for the past year. He had never had a steady girlfriend and had only once brought a girl home. 'And she was a real weirdo!' said his mother.

Gordon, however, was a model of convention. Good job, nice girlfriend, moderate drinker, sensible with money and soberly dressed in contrast with Mike's rather punk appearance, scruffy hair and earring. The initial session established the beginning of a potentially productive working relationship and also managed to reframe Mike's paranoia as shyness or uncertainty with strangers. They had asked their doctor to arrange a referral to a psychiatrist but now they suggested that they might prefer to wait and see how our next session went. Again it was the exploration of family relationships and background which provided one of the strongest indicators for a direction for the work with this family. The almost elderly appearance of the parents and the age difference between them – Mr Phillips was 64, fifteen years older than his wife – led me to ask directly whether Mike was their first-born child and how long they had been married before his birth. The warm way in which they related how much they had yearned for a baby over the first seven years of their marriage, their joy at Mike's arrival and his sensitive nature all combined to make him a very special child for them. Whilst Gordon looked a little bored with all this sentiment, Mike was enjoying every word, never having heard this story before. Questions about Mr and Mrs Phillips' own experience of growing up revealed that neither had left their parental home until they married. Mr Phillips had been an only child of doting and protective parents. Clearly separation was a topic on which their belief patterns were long established and fitted comfortably with each other. Questions around these beliefs revealed that the couple had planned to do some leisurely travel now that Mr Phillips had retired but they had abandoned this dream because they 'couldn't leave the boys'.

This suggested an overturn of the more traditional issues about leaving home and led to an intervention addressing the need for the parents to demonstrate to their sons that they no longer needed to be at home to ensure their parents' safety. The parents willingly agreed to go away for a weekend as an experiment following which there was a dramatic series of changes in the family. Mike found a job and soon afterwards a 'suitable' girlfriend. He became more confident, lost interest in drugs and began dressing more attractively. After three sessions, we agreed not to arrange further sessions but to see them if they wanted to contact us again. At follow-up a year or so later they were doing well.

(Seligman 1986)

Both these cases show that by exploring contexts, relationships, beliefs and background in a focused way within a systemic framework, change can be facilitated relatively speedily. For these young people and their families, there was possibility of long-term involvement either with the social services or the psychiatric network with the risk of labelling as 'bad' or 'mad'.

Of course, family therapists work with individuals and couples as well as with varying assortments of people who form systems.

Stephen was a 45-year-old man referred by his general practitioner. He was described as depressed and lacking in confidence and suffering from constant severe head pains for many years. Stephen confirmed this adding that his headaches had begun when he was 23 and at university. He recalled feeling a sort of explosion inside his head and had never been free of pain since. He was convinced that he had suffered some irreparable damage inside his head despite innumerable tests and examinations which detected nothing abnormal. The headaches, he explained, prevented him from leading a more successful life. He had had to take a year off work recently because it was impossible to concentrate and he was frequently overcome by lethargy. He had never been married but, for the past three years, had lived with a 23–year-old woman who had a history of depression and psychiatric disorder. 'She's a bit of a liability because we drag each other down', he said. 'But I'm afraid to lose her – I'm like an uncle to her and she needs me.'

Stephen's elderly parents had both died within the last few years and he felt, he said, 'both a loss and a sense of freedom'. In our first session he was surprised that I asked about his childhood but soon became enthusiastic about filling in a picture of a lonely and isolated only child of repressed and discouraging parents who never seemed to approve of anything he did. He had had no friends, no outside interests and from puberty he was beset by sexual fantasies which engendered terrible guilt in him and convinced him that he must be a bad and worthless person thus confirming what he suspected was his parents' view of him. I showed him the family tree I had drawn as he was talking – just three people, mother, father and son – and remarked that they looked very isolated as a family. Was he sure there were no other relations that he knew of? 'Oh, they had another baby but she died before I was born and they never spoke of her', he said casually. He saw no significance in this piece of information and was curious that I added the long-dead baby to the family tree. I asked him if he thought his parents might have still been grieving over their loss when he was born and if so, whether he thought that would have made any difference? He looked startled and uncomfortable and repeated that he hadn't even known about his sister's death until he was an adult. I waited quietly for a minute and then he said 'Mind you, I never felt I was quite what they wanted.'

At the end of the session he said he would like to come again. 'But do you think there really is something physical causing this headache? Can it be cured or is there some damage?' I looked grave as I said that I did indeed think there was a cause for his pain. His attention was riveted. 'I believe your sinuses are inflamed by unshed tears but I think it may need more than a nasal spray to deal with the inflammation, it may take a talking cure. I don't know it if will help but it's worth a try.' He fingered his forehead thoughtfully as he left.

Since this work is continuing at the time of writing, I still do not know if there will be a satisfactory outcome. However, Stephen has, for the first time, conceded that he might be cured and that life might improve for him. He is also beginning to accept that as a mature man, he might begin to challenge the beliefs instilled in his childhood and to reformulate his own beliefs without disloyalty to his parents' memory.

An example of therapy with a couple shows that extending the focus to include wider family, past generations and other professionals may not always suffice. Family systems overlap with a multiplicity of other systems including community and society with its political overtones. The ethical pros and cons involved in the therapist's own political views and how these are dealt with in the therapy relationship are complex but an awareness of how clients are affected by, for instance, gender role beliefs and the willingness to explore the implications of these can be crucial.

Martin and Elspeth were a professional couple living and working in Wales for a year or so. Their only daughter was at home in the USA completing her university degree. They sought help for their marriage relationship saying that there was so much despair and anger between them that they continually rowed and said hateful things to each other. Both described childhoods beset by difficulties and disturbing events and Martin had been in analytical therapy for nearly ten years up until eight or nine years ago. Ten years ago Elspeth had had a brief affair and despite Martin's denials, she was convinced that he still harboured a grievance against her. She confessed that she felt strong resentment that Martin had done all his confiding to his therapist (a male) which she had experienced as a long and intimate extra-marital relationship and 'worse than an affair – a betrayal'.

Each session went well but with few exceptions the couple returned with little change to report and I felt increasingly stuck. Each of them felt invalidated by the other and each saw themselves as a victim of the other's oppressive behaviour and so were constantly on guard against each other. The best they seemed to manage was an occasional armed truce. Then, one day, a conversation between them during a session highlighted what I thought of as a political issue around gender roles. I decided to share my thoughts with them saying that I wasn't sure if they'd think it was relevant but perhaps it may interest them. 'I think that you Elspeth have been thinking a lot about feminist ideas in the last few years and I believe that some of your rage is for yourself but some of it is for the centuries of oppressed women about whom you feel frustrated and powerless.' Elspeth had begun to weep quietly as I spoke and I continued 'You, Martin and Elspeth, are one of the many, many couples who are victims of history at a time of evolution. In a curious way, women who have very macho partners are better able to vent their rage – they have something to hit upon! But women whose partners are sympathetic to feminist ideas, as Martin is, have nowhere to resolve their rage. You are both victims of society and I fear it will take another two generations to change things.' They both had tears in their eyes. Clearly these ideas did have some relevance for them and the idea that they were both somehow trapped in a web for which they could not be blamed allowed them to comfort one another. From that session they were, at last, able to step back a little and to begin to work together for a more peaceful and harmonious relationship. Somehow the reframing of their situation gave them the opportunity to see themselves more objectively and as part of a wider system. They grasped at the opportunity and used it to nurture goodwill and to see the meaning of their previous struggles differently.

Over the past two decades a number of doubts and criticisms of family therapy have been expressed with varying degrees of effect. In the light of critiques from a number of directions, practice has continually evolved, as befits a theory which gives high priority to the concept of recursivity and which recognizes as significant the inter-connectedness between systems of all kinds from the individual to wider global systems. Much of the early criticism opposed family therapy because it was unfamiliar and therefore perceived as threatening to the more established way of approaching human problems. At first this opposition, along with charges that working in teams, often with one-way screens and video-recording, was both expensive and unethical, produced a response in some family therapists akin to a missionary zeal!

However, thankfully, there has been a considered response to the broad ethical questions around issues of potentially oppressive practice and misuse of power. As well as considering these issues in the client population, family therapists have looked, sometimes painfully, at their own practices. Clients are more often given opportunities to make real choices about teams, videos and even the choice of therapist (e. g. black or white, male or female) without being judged as 'difficult'. Clients' rights to be respected and therapists' recognition of potential power imbalances in the therapeutic relationship are widely discussed and acknowledged in training and are integrated into the Association for Family Therapy's code of ethics.

Questions such as how to define a family; do family therapists only try to keep families together; and are family therapists only seeing the easy cases while social workers are left to struggle on with heavy statutory work have, I believe, largely been answered. The notion of neutrality helps to prevent the therapist from pushing a family in one direction or another; the notion of systems disposes of the need to define a family – the relevant system is different from case to case; therapists (who may themselves have statutory responsibilities) often work in close collaboration with other professionals where these are seen as part of the client's relevant system.

Feminist approaches to practice and the issues of race and culture are dealt with in other chapters but it is important to include here a tribute to the influence of the feminist critique upon family therapy. Its effect has been crucial over the past ten years and there is a high awareness of the implications for practice of feminist thinking. Indeed, teaching about anti-discriminatory practices is incorporated on all training courses which are registered with the Association for Family Therapy.

NOTE

1   In May 1993 a register of psychotherapists was founded in the UK, and suitably qualified family therapists may apply for registration in order to be entitled to describe themselves as family psychotherapists.

REFERENCES

Barker, P. (1986) *Basic Family Therapy*, Glasgow: Collins.
Palazzoli, M. S. *et al.* (1978) *Paradox and Counter-Paradox*, Northvale, NJ: Aronson.
Seligman, P. M. (1986) 'A brief family intervention with an adolescent referred to drug taking', *Journal of Adolescence*, September.

FURTHER READING

Avis, J. (1989) 'Integrating gender into the family therapy curriculum', *Journal of Feminist Family Therapy* 2(3): 3–26.
Bodin, A. (1969) 'Family therapy training literature: a brief guide', *Family Process* 8(2): 272.
Boyd-Franklin, N. (1989) *Black Families in Therapy: A Multi-Systems Approach. Implications for Training and Supervision*, Woking, Surrey: Guildford Press.
Breunlin, D. C., Schwarz, R. C. and MacKune-Karrer, B. (1992) *Metaframeworks, Transcending the Models of Family Therapy*, San Francisco: Jossey-Bass.
Cade, B. W. and Seligman, P. M. (1982) 'Teaching a strategic approach', in R. Whiffen and J. Byng-Hall (eds) *Family Therapy Supervision, Recent Developments in Practice*, London: Academic Press.
Cade, B. W., Speed, B. and Seligman, P. M. (1986) 'Working in teams: the pros and cons', in F. W. Kaslow (ed.) *Supervision and Training: Models, Dilemmas and Challenges*, London: Haworth Press.
Ceccin, G. (1987) 'Hypothesizing, circularity and neutrality revisited: an invitation to curiosity', *Family Process* 26(4).
Coleman, S., Avis, J. and Turin, M. (1990) 'A study of the role of gender in family therapy training', *Family Process* 29(4).
Coyne, J. (1986) 'The significance of the interview in strategic marital therapy', *Journal of Strategic and Systemic Therapies* 5(1): 2.
Dimmock, B. and Dungworth, D. (1985) 'Beyond the family: using network meetings with statutory child care cases', *Journal of Family Therapy* 7(1): 45–68.
Furlong, M. and Scott, E. (1989) 'Can a family therapist do statutory work? The family, the statutory worker and the therapist working together for change', *The Australian and New Zealand Journal of Family Therapy* 10(4), p. 211.
Jones, E. (1987) 'Brief systemic work in a psychiatric setting where a family member has been diagnosed as schizophrenic', *Journal of Family Therapy* 9(1): 3–26.
Jones, E. (1992) *Working with Adult Survivors of Child Sexual Abuse*, London: Karnac Books.
Liddle, H., Breunlin, D. and Schwartz, R. (1988) *Handbook of Family Therapy, Training and Supervision*, Woking, Surrey: Guildford Press.
Lipchik, E. and De Shazer, S. (1986) 'The purposeful interview', *Journal of Strategic and Systemic Therapies* 5(1): 2.
O'Brian, C. and Bruggen, P. (1985) 'Our personal and professional lives. Learning positive connotation and circular questioning', *Family Process* 24(3): 311.
Penn, P. (1985) 'Feed-forward: Future questions future maps', *Family Process* 24(3): 299.
Roberts, J. (1988) 'Rituals and trainees', in E. Imber-Black, J. Roberts and R. Whiting (eds) *Rituals in Families and Family Therapy*, Farnborough, Hants: Norton Press.
Seligman, P. M. and Jones, E. (1987) *Systemic Family Therapy*, Video tape, Macmed Scotland.

Speed, B., Seligman, P. M., Kingston, P. and Cade, B. W. (1982) 'A team approach to family therapy', *Journal of Family Therapy* 4(3).

Storm, C. (1991) 'Placing gender in the heart of MFT Masters programmes', *Journal of Marital and Family Therapy* 17(1): 45–52.

Street, E. and Dryden, W. (1988) (eds) *Family Therapy in Britain*, Milton Keynes: Open University Press.

Tomm, K. (1987) 'Interventive interviewing: Part 1. Strategizing as a fourth guideline for the therapist', *Family Process* 26(1).

Whiffen, R. and Byng-Hall, J. (1982) (eds) *Family Therapy Supervision: Recent Developments in Practice*, London: Academic Press.

13 Welfare rights

Paul Burgess

There is hardly a family or individual in the UK whose quality of life is not in some degree affected by the income maintenance system. It accounts for over 30 per cent of government expenditure, and provides the most likely and the most enduring circumstances in which the individual will become engaged with a bureaucracy of the state. This is the broad subject matter of the activity known as welfare rights, which is concerned with the actual 'welfare rights' of individuals within this system. For many people it is a central aspect of their lives, because they are not able to work, or cannot earn enough, to keep them out of poverty. This may be because of unemployment, disablement, single parenthood, old age, or poverty wages. Benefits which are related to their low incomes, that is, means-tested benefits, are very important to them. But entitlements to many other types of pensions and benefits also extend, by virtue of national insurance contributions, or through the satisfaction of simple qualifying conditions, to many people who are not poor. However, the clients of social workers will, as a known fact, fall largely in the former category.

Some other facts are also important. The system of social security pensions and allowances, housing benefits, National Health Service charge exemptions, social services provisions, and education benefits, is complicated. It is based upon detailed Acts of Parliament and regulations, backed up with extensive guidance manuals for officials, and provided by an uncoordinated range of different official bodies, some of which are local and others national. And it is subject to constant change, with rules and policies being amended continuously. A critical problem is the change which occurs annually in the qualifying levels of entitlement, due mainly to the effects of inflation on money values. Consequently, vast quantities of leaflets and information materials have to be revised and re-issued. For the ordinary person the result can be an abundance of unreliable information, and for advisers there is the need to replace frequently their hard won familiarity with the various schemes, and the figures associated with them, and immediately re-acquire a professional competence with the new information.

Beyond the information and advice levels, which are vital to the public's access to the system, there are other areas where help is needed. Decisions based upon the judgement or discretion of officials are central to the adjudication process, and the applicant or claimant is often disadvantaged when questioning these decisions. For this reason experienced advisers provide a valuable service when they enter the discussions or negotiations on the side of the members of the public; they can ensure that vital facts are fully appreciated, or introduce a different perspective in the interpretation of the regulations, or simply identify mistakes. In addition, apart from the notorious exception of the Social Fund (where other less satisfactory avenues for appeal are provided) virtually every decision of officialdom in the field of benefits is open to challenge before an independent appeal tribunal, and the availability of skilled representation is often decisive in a successful appeal. Sometimes the problem is the way the matter has been handled by officialdom, and a point may be reached where injustice has been caused by maladministration and the only option left is to take the complaint to an ombudsman. Practical advice and help, such as the drafting of the submission, will be crucial for many if they are to have their grievance articulated in an effective way.

This, in a nutshell, is a description of the context in which welfare rights work takes place. It is a relatively new activity, even in relation to social work itself, having emerged from, and grown alongside, the development of an increasingly elaborate, and economically and socially important, structure of income maintenance provision. The question now is how it all relates to the social worker's role.

And the remarkable fact is that this takes us into controversial territory. It is a controversy which has been around, to my personal knowledge, for at least twenty years, and all the signs are that it will not go away. This is the issue: many social workers argue that they cannot be expected to provide their clients with help concerning their welfare rights, because (a) it is not their job, and (b) to attempt to do so will detract from the limited time and energy they have to give to the main duties and statutory responsibilities for which they are liable. There has been regular and persuasive argument to the contrary, and, in fact, many social workers demonstrate very effectively their acceptance of the obligation to help their clients with welfare rights problems. Cohen and Rushton (1982: 13), from a standpoint very sympathetic to the dilemmas facing social workers, enquire into the reasons for the reluctance to undertake welfare rights work. Their view is that 'the answer lies partly in lack of resources, partly in the fact that the agency may not give it priority and partly in differing views about the nature of social work'. Two particularly interesting points emerge from the thorough and fair treatment they give to the opposing arguments. Welfare rights work as advocacy may be seen as overt conflict and is therefore hard to cope with given the social worker's inclination to make good relationships. This may be true, but often it seems as though the reluctance lies not so much in the conflictual aspects of this activity, for surely social workers can hardly be strangers to conflict, but rather in the inclination to accept, unless there is overwhelming evidence of unfairness, that the official view is right, and their client's perception of the issue distorted or wrong. In this respect they share the naivety of much of the general public.

On the other hand, is welfare rights work compatible with the therapist/client model of social work? How can a commitment to rights and entitlements fit with subjective views and judgements about, for example, the client's motivation to find work (Cohen and Rushton 1982: 20)? A concern with perhaps more legitimacy, though still totally unacceptable from the welfare rights viewpoint, arises from the notion that obtaining certain benefits can result in the labelling of the client. Most often this is associated with the receipt of disability benefits, and it is sometimes shared with the medical profession who feel that emphasizing what a person *can't* do is unhelpful to their recovery. And there is an uncomfortably high incidence of ill-informed comment on the part of social workers concerning the wholly lawful and proper pursuit of entitlements by, for example, carers who must struggle with the system on behalf of both themselves and their dependants. Because of the grave inadequacies of the social security provision for carers we have a situation where although dependants are reliant upon carers for their personal needs, the carers become financially reliant upon the dependants' benefits; not surprisingly, this results in the integration of the carers' and dependants' interests.

A less accommodating and more combative approach to the issue is taken by Becker and MacPherson (1988). From outside social work it is rather difficult to see where the line can be drawn between helping a family with problems caused by factors such as poor housing, health, child care or family breakdown, and helping them to obtain better social security. But many would go further and insist that the analysis of social work must also reach into the roots of so much that is seen as personal weakness and inadequacy, and find the contribution which poverty itself is making. Tunnard (in Becker and MacPherson 1988: 129) reported that the families of the great majority of children in the care of local authorities in the 1980s were dependent upon the lowest incomes (that is supplementary benefit, now known as income support). Consequently, she concludes 'Social workers cannot be expected to make good the inadequacies of the welfare system. But as the job of social work is to cope with the casualties of poverty, the financial worries of clients cannot be ignored.'

The thrust of the argument based upon the poverty of clients must, nevertheless, be kept in proportion. It is *not* the same as saying that all poor people require the help of social workers, which is palpably untrue.

One of the difficulties for the non-social worker may be a proper view of the commitment which social workers can give to welfare rights work. Of course, social workers *must* have a basic knowledge of the benefits structure, and of course many of the problems clients have are related to the need for practical help and assistance, for which they should be able to turn to the social worker. But it is illusory to believe that social workers can, on the whole, do more than struggle inadequately with the increasingly sophisticated system in which their clients may be enmeshed. Unless, that is, they are provided with the resources, training and time they need. Even then, it is not clear whether the attempt should be to provide them with the full works, or simply to aim for a modest degree of efficiency in fulfilling their minimum obligations. For example, what is the best advice for someone who has just found a whopping underpayment in a client's benefit? Get a colleague to check it again with you. Many a well-intentioned social worker has been ruined for life by the full-measured scorn of a social security clerk who could add up better. And when is honesty with the client most important? When you don't know the answer. Wrong or misleading information is not only damaging to the client's immediate interests but is also, when it outs, as it most surely will, quite destructive of the social worker's credibility – and so it should be too.

In the attempt to avoid an active involvement with the welfare rights problems which clients face – and there does seem to be universal acceptance of the fact that clients have these problems, and that social workers face expectations that they will be able to help – a variety of defences are made. Some have merit, and it would be foolish not to see that in the enduring debate there is something difficult or fundamental at stake. Fimister (1986) has compiled the following comprehensive list together with a critical commentary:

1 Welfare rights work is not part of real social work.
2 Social workers should not strain relations with other official agencies.
3 Welfare rights work is too complex for the non-specialist.
4 Some other agency should handle welfare rights.
5 Computers should do it.
6 Welfare rights should concentrate on take-up campaigns which reach more people.
7 It is good for clients to do it for themselves.

Many of these points have legitimacy to varying degrees. In fact, most welfare rights commentators appreciate that, fundamentally, the argument is not that social workers should also be skilled welfare rights advisers, but that they should recognize that an effective response to the welfare rights problems of their clients is essential. That can mean different things in different cases. For example, if a client with child care problems has her income support payment stopped, and you know she is inarticulate and unable to write letters, can you ignore the impact this will have upon her family's circumstances and your work with her? Again, if you work with disabled people to increase their independence, or you must assess the need for domiciliary services, can you brush aside questions about entitlement to disablement benefits? Indeed, if charges for those services are to be contemplated, can this reasonably be undertaken without also giving relevant information about, and help with, claims for benefits?

The answers, surely, must be negative in each case. However, the difficulty is that apparently simple matters, which are within the competence of a reasonably well-informed person, can sometimes develop into more complex issues requiring more welfare rights knowledge and experience, and time, to deal with than the social worker possesses. It is then legitimate to look for help from specialist welfare rights advisers.

In this respect, some social workers and their clients will be more fortunate than others. The provision of welfare rights advisers, or more substantially, welfare rights services, although increasingly common, is still far from being widespread. As an activity welfare rights has an extremely short history, with its roots in the 'rediscovery' of poverty in the mid-1960s (specifically the publication by Abel-Smith and Townsend 1965), the attention given to welfare benefits from 1965 onwards by the newly formed Family Poverty Group – later to become the Child Poverty Action Group (McCarthy 1986: 42) – whose first secretary, Tony Lynes, moved on in 1969 to a post in Oxfordshire children's department where, until 1971, he operated as a welfare rights adviser in all but name (Fimister 1986: 47), and the climate for innovation in social services engendered by the Seebohm Report published in 1968. Indeed, it has been suggested that the introduction of the concept of generic social workers made the introduction of a benefit specialism a natural development, although I am bound to say there is also something inherently contradictory in this view (Berthoud *et al.* 1986: 12). This confluence of events (and with a branch of the Child Poverty Action Group active locally) was certainly behind the call by Manchester City Council, in February 1968, for a conference of the 'children's, welfare, housing, health and education departments immediately on receipt of the report of the Seebohm Committee', together with voluntary organizations, with the task of reporting on methods for

(1) the early detection of the effects of poverty in Manchester families
(2) the examination of the adequacy of existing arrangements for obtaining

assistance of all kinds and to make proposals for (a) ways and means of improving public awareness of entitlement to benefits and (b) improving existing methods of application for benefits and any recommendations for simplification of present procedures.

(Resolution of Manchester City Council, 7 February, 1968)

Since it is from these developments that the first local authority welfare rights service originated the history may be of interest. The conference met in February 1969, and spawned a working party whose first action was the launching, in September 1969, of a 'campaign to advise people about welfare benefits', which may have been the first local authority sponsored take-up campaign. Some 200,000 copies of a leaflet entitled 'These are your rights' were distributed to every household, and, significantly for our present purpose, a handbook on benefits was produced for social workers. The impact of the campaign was mixed (the leaflet's design left a lot to be desired) and when the conference met again in May 1971 the proposals which emerged were less ambitious and more specific; but they included the seminal proposal that the city 'should undertake a pilot scheme by appointing a welfare rights officer to operate in one area of the city and to investigate at grass roots level how people can best be informed about welfare benefits'.

Subsequently, the decision was taken that the post should be in the newly established social services department, and be located in the area with the highest referral rate for social work services. By the time I took up the post in August 1972 the job description also included the task of assessing the effectiveness of the methods used to publicize the services and benefits available. There was little notion in the department of what was actually needed, and so a process of investigation and discovery over several months led to a service giving direct advice and help to the public, with only a slight delay before representation at social security appeal tribunals was seen as an indispensable element of any self-respecting advice service. In retrospect the approach to this question by the social services senior management was curiously circumspect, although it should be borne in mind that it was not until 1975 that the National Association of Citizens Advice Bureaux came off the fence and decided they could represent clients at tribunals.

Because of the location in a social services area office it was also inevitable that the job would involve a consultancy to the social workers and their clients, though I was not prepared for the mountain of case files which appeared on my desk one day as 'referrals' – an experience that was not repeated. The wider implications of the advocacy aspects, particularly as they related to the local authority's own activities, were barely considered. Lynes, drawing on his own earlier experience, and the ruminations of a welfare rights officer in post for all of three weeks, was quick to see the key issues, and, bearing in mind the anxiety about the welfare rights advocacy implications since local authorities assumed full responsibility for community care in April 1993, may also have been prophetic:

> The inevitable question posed by an appointment of this kind is, to what extent can or should a local government official permit his role to spill over from impartial advice to advocacy? How far will a welfare rights officer be allowed to go in doing battle with other departments – housing and education in particular – of the authority that employs him? For that matter, what will happen should he ever wish to act as advocate against the social services department? The answers to questions of this kind will decide whether Paul Burgess is the first of a new race of local government welfare-advocates or just an information officer.
>
> (Lynes 1972)

These questions served to set a challenging agenda, and certainly proved relevant in time both in relation to advocacy work with individuals and on policy issues. A report on the first nine months of the project concluded it had met successfully an important need, while revealing the extent of the unfairness and bureaucracy faced by poor people. The need for a multi-layered strategy was also recognized, with a personal service to the public married to publicity and take-up activities, and policy work attempting to influence central government and legislation (Burgess 1973). By 1974 a fully fledged welfare rights unit of five staff, with a publicity and take-up budget, became a permanent feature of the social services department (Manchester Social Services Department 1975).

With the initiative in Manchester apparently acting as a catalyst, in 1974 no less than ten other local authorities appointed full-time welfare rights staff, followed by an average of two authorities a year until 1981; the following four years saw some thirty-five new teams established, largely as a response to the trebling of unemployment to 3,000,000 between 1980 and 1981. In 1986, when a comprehensive survey was undertaken, around sixty-five local authorities had a welfare rights provision of some kind (Berthoud *et al.* 1986: 8). An additional consideration has been the recognition that despite reductions in local authorities' subsidies by central government, efforts aimed at increasing the take-up of social security benefits, which are central government funded, can have a directly beneficial impact upon household incomes and thus the local economy.

Since then there has been further growth in provision, with debt counselling emerging as a new and important area of need. Occasionally, new resources have been provided in partnership schemes with advice agencies outside the local authority. Nevertheless, recently in a small number of dramatic instances political changes have led to the abandonment of services

– most notably in Bradford, in Yorkshire, although the 1991 local elections reversed the situation and the first steps in rebuilding the service have been taken. The current bleak financial situation for local government produced by the poll tax, and now the council tax, suggests that the opportunities for local authorities to introduce new services in the near future will simply not be available, unless spending can be switched from existing budget provision.

The relationship between full-time welfare rights services within a local authority and the social services department, or, more narrowly, the social workers within that department, varies considerably. A major factor influencing the relationship is the location of the welfare rights service itself; although most are to be found within the structure of the social services department, a significant minority are part of the chief executive's department (Berthoud *et al.* 1986: 21). Another factor is the provision of a direct welfare rights advice service to the public; where this is an important part of the structure of the service, social workers and their clients are usually (in theory) required to take their place in the queue, rather than being given privileged access to the welfare rights officers. Where referrals are contemplated, great emphasis is placed upon the concept of a negotiated referral, which obliges the social worker to make contact and discuss the nature of the client's problem before referring to the welfare rights service. Apart from ensuring that they can actually help, the purpose is also to focus on the degree of information and practical help which the social worker may be able, on reflection, to provide from available resources. Where the service does not offer direct personal help to the public the alternative model is usually a welfare rights consultancy for social workers and others, often with firm in-house training commitments.

However, these are the two extremes, and more commonly a mixture of activities is found including, in addition, policy and benefits take-up work. In Lancashire, for example, where a welfare rights service was introduced into the chief executive's department in 1987, in addition to the provision of a service of information, advice, and tribunal representation to the public from county-wide free-standing town centre locations, and local consultancy and training for other professionals and organizations, there is also a take-up and publicity unit which fills gaps in the range of official information and runs high-profile campaigns each year, and information, training and research activities located centrally. The existence of the service is also represented in the political structures through a welfare rights subcommittee of the county council's policy and resources committee, and this enables not only service questions to be addressed by members but also policy issues concerning the impact on the county's citizens of government action and other matters arising out of the income maintenance system. In total some forty-nine staff are employed in the service, around 60,000 enquiries a year are dealt with at the local offices, of which four out of ten need follow-up work, often including eventual representation at a variety of appeal tribunals. To give these figures some perspective, the county's population is 1.4 million, and in 1992–3 approximately £2 billion will be received by residents as income from pensions and benefits of various kinds, that is, almost 25 per cent of domestic household income.

There is no question that a welfare rights service of this kind, which deals frequently with money entitlements of considerable significance (entailing thousands of pounds annually for thousands of people) as well as the deep, personal sense of a right to just and fair treatment of thousands more, must be professionally and efficiently delivered; but it is also essential that its values are absolutely clear. The response to the request for help must be geared to providing independent advice and practical help directly related to the needs and best interests of *each* of the service's customers, while ensuring that their dignity and self-respect is safeguarded by enabling them, once properly resourced, to secure their rights by their own efforts as far as possible. Often there is an unavoidable tension in this position between effective action and control by the customer, but each case is unique.

Space does not allow a full treatment of the various elements and emphases to be found in different welfare rights services around the country, but they have usually been the driving force behind issues such as improving the delivery of local authority benefits services by integrating the administration of housing benefits and education welfare benefits, and the analysis and implementation of authority-wide policies dealing with poverty. Many play a part in the structuring (and in some instances the rescuing!) of community care projects, and other social services schemes, and literally millions of pounds have been generated as a result of advice and consultancy roles. The raising of the profile of advice activities, both within local authorities and outside, and through community-based provision, is also an objective and a product. Developing information technology applications for both advisory purposes and computer-based targeted take-up campaigns and projects has been a persistent theme, especially over the last decade, with considerable success being achieved. Furthermore, the design and publication of good publicity and information materials has evidently been a major influence on the standards aimed for by government departments, with the emphasis on plain English being a noticeable achievement. And, finally, improvements in the benefits system are frequently sought through efforts directed at changing and improving government policies; efforts which are necessary because of the knowledge we have of the day-to-day injustice and unfairness experienced by many of our customers.

Much of this activity leads, in those local authorities where there are welfare rights services provided, to an increase in the help accruing to social workers and their clients, either through direct and tangible improvements in the departmental support and liaison achieved or through the overall attention given to benefits issues. There is no reason to suppose that this would not continue. However, during the relatively short existence of welfare rights services there has been an enormous degree of change in their environment, and all the signs are that this will be undiminished in the future. And more than most services they have been under the spotlight, and needing to justify that existence. Largely this is because of the visible impact of their activities, but it is also because their work is perceived as politically sensitive. One unsung achievement in this respect is the part they have played in the dramatic conversion of the Department of Social Security, during its conversion into the new Benefits Agency, to real information and advice services to its customers (the word claimant has been dropped) as opposed to its token approach in the past. Although there is still a very long way to go before many of its customers will trust the advice given (and *can* trust it – at present much of it should carry a financial health warning) there seems no doubt that more than the vocabulary has changed, and that the changes are very much in concert with the criticisms made by welfare rights services over many years. How they themselves will need to respond to the new situation remains to be seen, but I cannot see that the Benefits Agency can meet, even with computer-aided 'one-stop information' strategies, either the public's need for advice and advocacy which is underpinned by the fundamental values referred to above, or, and as a direct consequence, the level of professional all-round welfare rights competence required.

Finally, as welfare rights as a professional activity moves into its third decade, it may be that its proper place in the spectrum of legal services provision in the UK will be established. For the reality is that most of the time, and from the very beginning (Cohen and Rushton 1982: 5), the professional welfare rights adviser has functioned in a role equivalent to a lawyer, and there are few obvious similarities with social work. True, the concern is with 'welfare' law, and social services departments originally brought them forth into the world, but the tendency has been for welfare rights work to differentiate increasingly between social services positions and its own. The proposed reforms in the use of the Legal Aid scheme, which see a wider range of agencies other than solicitors having access to the Legal Aid to finance the legal work they do, may act as the final point of departure in this regard. In order to meet the assured quality standard it is vital that the agency can demonstrate not only a legal competence but also the integrity and independence of its personal advisory services, and this may only be possible if the accountability to social services managers of many welfare rights advisers is ended.

Of course, if this materializes, it should not mean the end of the expectations upon social workers, with which this chapter began, to help and assist their clients where the need is proportionate to the social worker's abilities and resources. Who knows, it may even serve to reiterate the obligation created by the exclusiveness of the relationship with the client?

REFERENCES

Abel-Smith, B. and Townsend, P. (1965) *The Poor and the Poorest*, London: Bell.
Becker, S. and MacPherson, S. (eds) (1988) *Public Issues, Private Pain*, London: Insight.
Berthoud, R., Benson, S. and Williams, S. (1986) *Standing up for Claimants: Welfare Rights Work in Local Authorities*, London: Policy Studies Institute.
Burgess, P. (1973) 'Rights man in welfare', *New Society*, 13 September.
Cohen, R. and Rushton, A. (1982) *Welfare Rights*, London: Heinemann Educational Books/*Community Care*.
Fimister, G. (1986) *Welfare Rights Work in Social Services*, London: Macmillan.
Lynes, T. (1972) 'Welfare men', *New Society*, 14 September.
McCarthy, M. (1986) *Campaigning for the Poor: CPAG and the Politics of Welfare*, London: Croom Helm.
Manchester Social Services Department (1975) *Report: Development of the Welfare Rights Service in the City of Manchester*, September.

FURTHER READING

Baldwin, S., Parker, G. and Walker, R. (1988) *Social Security and Community Care*, Aldershot: Avebury.
Freeman, M. D. A. (ed.) (1990) *Critical Issues in Welfare Law*, London: Steven and Sons.
Hemming, R. (1984) *Poverty and Incentives: The Economics of Social Security*, Oxford: Oxford University Press.
Millar, J. (1989) *Poverty and the Lone Parent Family*, London: Avebury.
Walker, R. and Parker, G. (1988) *Money Matters: Income, Wealth, and Financial Welfare*, London: Sage.

14 Written agreements : a contractual approach to social work

Michael Preston-Shoot

What is a contract? Consider the following agreement involving a mother and child, a residential establishment where they were living, and a social services department contemplating care proceedings.

> Contract between Social Services, Green House and Beatrice Brown.
> This eight-week period will assess Ms Brown's:
>
> 1 mothering and parenting skills;
> 2 commitment to Robert, for example keeping to routines, seeing to his needs first, before her own, not forgetting about him;
> 3 emotional response and attachment to Robert (beyond bonding);
> 4 handling of the baby, Robert, and her ability to cope with him when he is crying and unhappy.
>
> This assessment must show beyond doubt that Ms Brown can cope with Robert on her own for a full day and night, and is able to take responsibility for caring for a baby with minimum support.
>   If the assessment does not conclude this, Ms Brown will not be allowed to take Robert home with her, and further proceedings will be taken. If for any reason staff at Green House feel that the baby is in danger, or is unsafe staying with his mother, the baby will be removed, social services informed, and the placement terminated.
>
> Signed............

What are your views about this written agreement? In particular, how far towards partnership does this agreement go, how much power and authority do the various participants have, and is Ms Brown likely to feel empowered? You might also consider what power and authority workers and service users need to work together effectively, and what agreement you would seek to negotiate in this situation.

Social work is a complex undertaking. Besides familiar practice dilemmas (Braye and Preston-Shoot 1992a) such as care versus control; rights versus risks; and needs versus resources, it can present conflicts between professional judgement and agency policy. It can involve conflicting views within a family or group, or between them and practitioners. Disagreements between users and workers about targets for change and/or how to achieve them can originate in workers' assumptions about needs, class, poverty, gender and problem-solving; or from users experiencing 'clienthood' as a state while workers perceive it as a transition (Phillimore 1982). Social work frequently involves anxiety in the face of chaotic situations, together with choices about where to intervene, how, when and with whom. Many users are victims of oppression and inequalities, yet services frequently individualize users' problems rather than challenge the social attitudes and structures in which discrimination is rooted.

Agreements or contracts, and the process of exchange of views which precedes them, may assist practitioners to contain anxiety and retain direction, to minimize misunderstanding, and to counter some of the negative effects of being service users (Corden and Preston-Shoot 1988). This is because they utilize key ingredients for successful work, namely:

1 Clearly defined problems, with specific objectives and tasks which are precise enough to provide a clear and agreed focus.
2 Openness and honesty, with differences of opinion and the power imbalance between user and worker openly addressed, and with the work's purposes clearly understood.
3 The active support of significant people in the user–worker environment.
4 User involvement in problem definition, decision making and reviews to ensure continuing relevance and clarity of the work.
5 User access to information and complaints procedures, to promote informed understanding and consent, and accountability.

Agreements form a basis for structuring interactions in which one or more intervention methods might be used, and for negotiating which methods are appropriate. Such is their wide applicability across different settings and methods that skill in using written agreements is now a basic competency for practitioners (CCETSW 1991).

Professional intervention can have depressing outcomes and potential side-effects: insufficient inter-professional communication (DHSS 1974; Goodman Report 1990; BCCCS 1991); inadequate planning and regulation (Levy and Kahan 1991); over-zealous use of statutory powers (Butler-Sloss 1988); disempowerment, mystification, dependence and users' loss of control to tackle problems effectively (Illich 1975; Smale 1983). Intervention can undermine individuals and their existing networks, and impose on them values of an oppressive and discriminatory society, for instance in relation to gender and family. Organizational policies and procedures can reflect structural inequalities and oppressive stereotypes, and a patronizing, colonizing, non-participative and unaccountable use of power and authority (Barclay 1982; Croft and Beresford 1989). Recent evidence of abuses in residential care highlights that organizational systems can exacerbate difficulties experienced by users.

There is a growing need to develop tools which challenge powerlessness, dependency, passivity and oppression (Lee 1991), which alter rather than work within existing power relationships and traditional definitions of need and agency responsibilities, and which recognize that organizational policies and attitudes may be targets for change. Moreover, involving users in decision making and transferring power to them generates a wide range of options which counter the negative effects of previous intervention and reduce the need for protective statutory intervention (Wilcox *et al.* 1991). These options include social change goals – taking action to address structures of oppression, exclusion, isolation and powerlessness arising from internalized oppression (Barber 1991; Mullender and Ward 1991).

When consideration is given to how negotiation and decision making is affected by race, gender and power (Mistry and Brown 1991; Phillipson 1992), using written agreements can convey respect, enhance user self-esteem, empower users to gain greater control over their lives (Maluccio and Simm 1989) and replace the voice of the expert with that of the oppressed (Dominelli 1988). The approach opens possibilities of learning from users and working in non-hierarchial ways (Hanmer and Statham 1988), for avoiding unwarranted intervention (DoH 1991a) and providing effective services (DoH 1989), for redressing the balance of power by promoting users' rights and skills to negotiate about their involvement (Corden and Preston-Shoot 1987b; DoH 1991b) and for engaging in relationships which emphasize partnership and professionals' accountability to users.

Finally, the requirements of social work law also promote a contractual approach to practice. The Children Act 1989 emphasizes working in partnership with children and parents. This applies whether the local authority is providing services to children in need, accommodating children, investigating child abuse, or working with children in care. The emphasis on partnership includes a requirement for written plans for children being looked after (DoH 1991c). These must be completed after consultation with children, parents and significant others, and be reviewed regularly. The arrangements specified in the plans *must* be agreed between the local authority and a person with parental responsibility (or the young person if aged 16 or over) if the child is accommodated, and *should* preferably be agreed for children in care, thus constituting a written agreement (Braye and Preston-Shoot 1992b). Written agreements can be between the local authority and people with parental responsibility; the local authority and a child; the local authority and foster carers and/or other agencies.

Guidance following the NHS and Community Care Act 1990 also emphasizes partnership between users and providers. This includes users being fully informed of the purpose of assessment and fully involved in decision making (Social Services Inspectorate 1991), having a written statement of the assessment outcome, and having a written care plan (DoH 1991d) where assessment of need is followed by service provision.

WHAT IS A WRITTEN AGREEMENT?

A contract is an agreement which binds the parties. Social work contracts are not legally binding agreements but are morally binding obligations, the outcome of discussion and negotiation.

There is a legal framework of rules governing legal contracts in law which may also be transferred to social work (Corden 1980; Corden and Preston-Shoot 1987a). This framework distinguishes between offer, acceptance, consideration, and intention.

Offer and acceptance do not have to be made in writing. When one party makes an offer, the other party must not only accept it, but also communicate that acceptance before the other party can be expected to consider themselves bound by an agreement.

Preceding an offer is an 'invitation to treat'. This allows a party to state their concerns and/or resources, and to encourage the other party to indicate their intentions, without necessarily making a commitment formally to engage or provide goods or services.

Consideration involves providing or promising to provide some goods, services, actions, or to refrain from actions which might damage the other party's interests. Excluded are any considerations given before the bargain was struck and any consideration which the party was bound by law to carry out. Thus, in social work contracts, the user or practitioner agreeing to visit weekly would be insufficient as a consideration if this visiting frequency was already required by law.

There must also be an 'intention to contract'. When using contracts in social work, people may 'sign' an agreement without intending that they be held to its terms. Great care needs to be taken to ensure that users (or workers from other agencies) realize that, in making a particular agreement, practitioners intend to implement it and abide by its terms. Equally essential is that the parties are willing and have the resources to tackle the problems and objectives specified.

A contract will be void if it was agreed in circumstances where one party was under duress (physical violence, threat of violence, threat of punishment). Undue influence is where one party, by virtue of the nature of their relationship, dominates the other. If the relationship is abused, the contract negotiated in such circumstances is voidable. This requires a focus on power and process. How free have users been to articulate their needs, aims and wishes, and not to be overwhelmed by the advice of practitioners or by their knowledge of what the worker wants? Incapacity relates to people who might be considered as in need of protection from exploitation. They can enter into agreements but, in the event of a dispute, the onus would be on the responsible party to demonstrate that the agreement and the services being offered were suitable to the other party's requirements.

Contracts can be ended in a variety of ways:

1   Both parties fulfil their side of the bargain; their joint aims are achieved, no further work is necessary, and the contract expires.
2   The agreement is unsuccessful. Both parties agree to release each other from their obligations and to cease working together, or renegotiate it to overcome the problems they have encountered.
3   Circumstances change dramatically such that the contract is no longer relevant. In this situation it has been *frustrated* and neither party can 'sue' the other.
4   One party fails to perform their side of the agreement. The other party may choose either to regard that failure as releasing them from their part of the agreement, or to seek a remedy.

A distinction may also be made between types of contract. The primary contract is that between worker and user. Secondary contracts are negotiated between worker/user and those others whose co-operation is required to ensure that the aims of the primary contract are achieved.

Preliminary – Interim – Mainstream – Disengagement in contracts refers to degrees of involvement between practitioners and users. Clarity of objectives and trust to establish the feasibility of working together can take time to evolve. Thus, a preliminary contract will cover the earliest stages of the work, perhaps an assessment or early work while other issues are being explored. An interim agreement is where the issues are becoming clearer and a commitment to work in some areas exists and must begin, but full agreement is not yet achieved. A mainstream agreement is a contract for the work, issues having been explored, aims agreed, and tasks confirmed. Disengagement refers to agreements where, with the work completed or almost finished, but where immediate closure might be regarded as unhelpful, a contract is negotiated which scales down gradually the contact between the parties.

Mutual and Reciprocal refer to the extent to which there is complete agreement on the issues to be tackled and the means by which this will be done (mutual) and to situations where the goals of the parties may differ but where there is sufficient common ground that they feel able to commit themselves to working towards achieving each other's aims.

Service contracts involve workers and users. Contingency contracts are agreements between two parties (such as parents and children) where workers help them with the negotiation.

The framework of a contractual agreement should include:

1 Venue, frequency and time of contacts.
2 Duration of agreement, and what will happen at the end of that time (transfer, closure, review and renegotiation).
3 Change in circumstances which would require variation, review or termination.
4 How a breakdown of the agreement might be dealt with.
5 What happens if someone is absent for a session; a crisis occurs; someone fails to deliver their part of the bargain; or other such eventualities.
6 The context in which the work is taking place (court orders, statutory duties, non-negotiable obligations).
7 Arrangements regarding recording and confidentiality.
8 Complaints procedures.
9 Arrangements for reviews: when, where, with whom (parents, children, significant others involved), about what (reconsider agreement and plan, consider legal issues, promote and safeguard welfare).

The substance of a contract is:

1 A statement of aims and objectives. Only realistic aims, framed positively not negatively, which are agreed or accepted by the other party should be stated.
2 Specific tasks/work needed to achieve these aims.
3 A clear statement of what each party is responsible for and is offering over and above their legal duties as citizen/officer of the local authority.
4 What intervention approaches or methods of work will be used; who should be present; what people will do if they/others are going to be absent; basic ground rules for meetings.
5 What would constitute breakdowns of the agreement and how these will be dealt with.

Children Act guidance and regulations (DoH 1991c) require that written agreements contain, so far as practicable, aims and plans for the child based on identified needs (including race and culture, health and education); how these needs will be met; aims, and timescale for the plan; support arrangements for the placement; visiting and review arrangements; contact arrangements for the child with family members and important others; other services to be provided; 'what if' arrangements in the event of placement breakdown; circumstances in which the child might be removed from the placement; requirements to notify changes in circumstances.

Community care plans following assessment of need (section 47, NHS and Community Care Act 1990) should contain (DoH 1991d) objectives; criteria for evaluating their achievement; the services to be provided and by whom; the cost to the user and agencies; other options considered; differences of opinion; unmet needs with reasons; responsibility for monitoring and review; dates of review.

THE CRITIQUE

Recent legislation in adult services and child care requires enabling and protective powers and duties to be implemented where possible in partnership with users and their families or carers. Written agreements form a central element in this partnership. However, some legislation is enabling, designed to challenge discrimination (Race Relations Act 1976), to foster partnership (Children Act 1989), or to promote participation in assessment, service design and delivery (Disabled Persons Act 1986; NHS and Community Care Act 1990). Other legislation is repressive – immigration controls, social security provisions, and enactments on sexual preference being examples (Braye and Preston-Shoot 1992a). Even where legislation is enabling, it is inconsistent in the degrees of user involvement promoted, muddled in the principles or priorities inspiring it, and unclear how competing perspectives between users and their families/carers should be resolved (Braye and Preston-Shoot 1992a, b).

Using contracts has also been viewed as oppressive (Rojek and Collins 1987), arising from the imposition of white Eurocentric norms and/or unachievable standards of parenting in child protection cases, or the failure to include structural issues, such as poverty and racism, in problem definition and change strategies. By ignoring the context in which users live and workers practise, written agreements become a tool of surveillance and coercion, a form of social control (Nelken 1987). Indeed, CCETSW (1991) promotes their use to clarify expectations of parenting behaviour and the consequences of their not meeting a child's basic needs. Practitioners control the agenda and compliance is demanded within assumed agreement on dominant values by which society is organized. The individual and the socio-political are divorced. Ideologies and social structures are not questioned (Rees 1991).

Oppression may arise also from undue influence: users are not free agents with wide room for choice or manoeuvre; practitioners have access to power and authority arising from resources, knowledge, language, training, agency position and statute. The sanctions available to users (ombudsperson; complaints procedures; judicial review) which would scrutinize decision making are less immediately accessible than those available to workers (breach; case closure; use of law). Even if this does not deter users, the extent to which intention and consent, because of the imbalance of power, can be inferred or assumed must be questionable. The double jeopardy is of 'as if' agreements and of 'outside' assessors not questioning the use of power or the impact of oppression on negotiations because of the existence of an agreement.

That contracts have been used as tools of social control should not surprise. The conflicting imperatives and practice dilemmas, endemic in social work practice and emanating from its legal and organizational context, create role ambiguity and insecurity (Preston-Shoot and Agass 1990), and inspire defensive practice (Braye and Preston-Shoot 1992a). Indeed, the organizational context of statutory agencies in which most practitioners operate is a major obstacle to empowering users. The importance of independent advocacy structures (Mullender 1991) arises partly because users' needs and rights lead them to question the services of which social workers are a part.

PRACTICE PRINCIPLES

A step-by-step model for negotiating, implementing and reviewing written agreements has been described elsewhere (Corden and Preston-Shoot 1987a). However the critique highlights particular ideas with which to make a difference at individual and organizational levels. The themes of power, empowerment and partnership underpin the values and skills for negotiating and using contracts within an anti-oppressive framework.

Values

Values shape beliefs, observations and practice. Consequently, if contracts and services are to reflect partnership and anti-oppressive practice, practitioners must appraise how individual and organizational values affect work. Otherwise social constructions and internalized values will permeate practice, with workers unable to challenge assumptions around which individuals structure their lives, or the constructions organizations place on family life, gender, caring, race and mental health (Preston-Shoot and Agass 1990). Constructing services based on partnership and anti-oppressive principles involves addressing the marginalization of users by service providers and society. This includes challenging stereotyping and monoculturalism, negative labelling and pathologizing, professional mystique, and the creation of dependency. It requires constant analysis of personal history and cultural inheritance in the form of attitudes, beliefs and principles (Francis 1988;

Stratton *et al.* 1990) and how these might reinforce existing power structures and assumptions.

When working with users, partnership demands critical appraisal of the use of power and authority: what power can practitioners transfer to users and how? How does the exercise of power and authority empower and disempower users? Altering the power imbalance also involves challenging internalized oppression, particularly by recognizing users' skills, abilities, strengths and resources (Mullender and Ward 1991) and by using groups to extend their networks of support and to provide opportunities to take up issues and pursue social change (Barclay 1982; Barber 1991).

Partnership and anti-oppressive practice suggest a tripartite debate between workers, users and managers on the work. How are the personal and the political, structural disadvantage and oppression and its impact, to be connected, defined and addressed? How might social work move beyond an individual focus towards social change? How are users' experiences to be heard and how might agencies take up their agendas?

Anti-oppressive practice skills

Practice which assumes oppression and restricted choices (Hanmer and Statham 1988) must open up the process of negotiation, by:

1 Asking to what extent must the agenda be controlled by worker and agency, whether framework (venue and frequency of meetings, procedures) or substance (objectives, content)? Are power and authority being used to assume compliance with particular values and procedures, or to enable users to challenge how issues are defined and to maximize their control over change efforts (Rees 1991)? This means clarifying the level of partnership offered, from involvement and consultation in decision-making processes within pre-determined limits controlled by service providers, through collaboration in defining issues and options, to user control (Pugh and De'Ath 1989). This involves clarifying what is or is not negotiable in terms of agency function/statutory duties.

2 Protecting users' rights and facilitating their entry into partnership by using the different types of agreement available, by engaging in preparatory work, and ensuring access to independent advice and advocates. Preparatory work (an 'invitation to treat') recognizes that users should not be expected to immediately and unwarily embrace partnership. Defensiveness is not necessarily a symptom of unco-operativeness. Fears, past experiences and expectations must be acknowledged and explored. Workers must also share why they believe a contractual approach is helpful, and discuss the power and authority which each participant has. Continual

monitoring should follow. How safe do users experience the negotiating space, for instance to challenge or to raise anxieties? How might racism or sexism, for instance, have influenced the process and what can be done to overcome this? Are safeguards built into the negotiating process for users and are they felt to be easy to use?

3 Not assuming disempowering levels of control or responsibility. This requires self-questioning about how workers share power (language used, information given, rationale for the approach discussed, understanding and intention ensured), and what power and control users perceive themselves to have. Practitioners must address any pressures users may feel to comply with workers' suggestions or to remain silent in the face of unfairness, and must negotiate rather than assume invited roles, for example 'expert'.

4 Sharing information and knowledge to make oppression and its effects visible (Dominelli 1988), to challenge personal blame and pessimism, and to enable users to acquire skills and identify opportunities to challenge their powerlessness, isolation and hopelessness (Rees 1991). This means extending practice beyond individual work to groupwork and community action (Barber 1991; Mullender and Ward 1991). Where experiences of oppression have been internalized, users may not believe that they can reclaim control over life events or exercise influence to achieve desired goals. Work to achieve this belief may be a necessary precursor or a parallel process to work on identified goals. People become committed, both to task and process, when they believe the work to be worthwhile in terms of effort and time, when they can expect success and when they value that success.

5 The emphasis must be on process as well as task. If processes in relationships are ignored, written agreements (and indeed social work itself) will fail and/or be experienced as oppressive (doing to, not working with). The skills of engaging, sensitivity, responsiveness, anticipating, exploring experiences and ideas, and understanding how previous relationships may affect present interactions are crucial. Deciding upon methods of work in relation to target objectives can only follow from seeking information and developing understanding about issues faced.

6 Questioning how interventions will be perceived and what messages or assumptions workers may be communicating, for example in relation to race and culture or gender and power, in defining problems and deciding targets for change.

7 Ensuring objectives are specific, relevant and realistic. Written agreements should clearly state how participants will assess movement towards objectives. Responsibilities must be clearly allocated and timescales realistic for the objectives agreed. Before finalizing agreements, con-

straints on change must be considered: is agency support available? Are important significant others (family, organizations) engaged in the change effort? What are the possible implications of the targetted change for those involved, and are the resources and potential gains stronger than possible losses or threats?

8 Emphasizing the 'rewards' for successful outcomes, not merely the sanctions for non-fulfilment. When breakdowns occur, those involved should not simply attribute blame to users but, especially, analyse the contribution of the professional system (Preston-Shoot and Agass 1990) and distinguish whether revision arises from disagreement over objectives and/or from divergence over the means to achieve these targets. Change is rarely completed at the first attempt. At the very least consolidation will be necessary. Relapses and change call for analysis and renegotiation, particularly of restraining forces on change.

Among possible criticisms of the contract quoted earlier are that it does not fulfil the criteria for agreements, being rather a set of instructions imposed on Ms Brown with sanctions for 'failure' and without any statement of what the workers were prepared to offer to achieve particular objectives. The power imbalance is left undisturbed. It is coercive rather than a partnership as envisaged by the Children Act. It fails to establish explicitly the standards of parenting being used, their relevance and feasibility, nor does it define the criteria by which the success of the intervention will be gauged. The sanctions available to Ms Brown are not specified, nor are her strengths and skills recognized. Her socio-economic context is omitted entirely, yet this might limit her room for manoeuvre or have culminated in internalized oppression.

The following agreement was negotiated following the principles outlined above.

Contract between Susan, Mr and Mrs Aubrey and ... Social Services Department.

Background
Susan is 7, the oldest of three children. Until recently she lived with her maternal aunt and uncle (Mr and Mrs A). This was an informal arrangement within the family. The two younger children remained with their mother. Care orders were obtained. Anne (mother) applied for revocation of the orders. However, before the case could be heard she received a custodial sentence.

Mr and Mrs Aubrey applied for a residence order (Section 8, Children Act 1989) in respect of all three children. This was supported by Anne but opposed by the local authority. Since they had not been placed together in foster care, with the agreement of all the parties, the court dealt first with Susan's case. A residence order was not granted. The court decided that Susan should live with Mr and Mrs Aubrey for a six-month trial period, after which decisions would be made regarding all three children. Susan remains subject to a care order, as do her siblings (Section 31, Children Act 1989).

Reason for placement
As directed by the court.

Aim of the placement
To assess the possibility of Susan being rehabilitated to the long-term care of Mr and Mrs Aubrey.

Who will do what, when and how to achieve this aim
 1 The local authority and Mr and Mrs Aubrey will work in partnership.
 2 Jayne (social worker) will meet with Susan at three-weekly intervals, but more frequently if requested or required, to talk about how Susan sees her future.
 3 Jayne will meet with Mr and Mrs Aubrey fortnightly, to discuss Susan's future. An early task will be to clarify the criteria by which the local authority will assess whether Susan can be rehabilitated.
 4 Jayne will liaise with schools, clinical psychologist, and siblings' foster parents to monitor the effect of rehabilitation upon (i) Susan (ii) Susan and siblings (iii) siblings.
 5 Mr and Mrs Aubrey will be offered consultation with a psychologist of their choice to be given independent advice on how to manage Susan's more extreme behaviour (aggression, temper tantrums, screaming).
 6 Mr and Mrs Aubrey will have day-to-day responsibility for Susan.
 7 Mr and Mrs Aubrey will financially support Susan.
 8 Mr and Mrs Aubrey will encourage Susan to join neighbourhood activities.
 9 Mr and Mrs Aubrey will supervise and monitor contact between Susan and Anne. Anne will work in co-operation with them and the local authority to positively promote Susan's welfare.
10 Jayne and Mr and Mrs Aubrey give permission to Susan to talk about problems with whomsoever she feels comfortable.

Arrangements for child within placement
 1 To be registered with GP and dentist, to have a medical, to have regular dental check-ups.
 2 To attend primary school regularly.
 3 To see a child psychologist monthly to monitor progress.

Contact arrangements
1 With siblings, once per week with aunt and uncle at social services, once per week with siblings in foster home, once every three weeks with siblings and social worker.
2 With mother, at the discretion of Mr and Mrs Aubrey, but not to have overnight contact unless accompanied by them.
3 Mr and Mrs Aubrey will inform the local authority if Susan is to be away from home for more than two nights.
4 Susan may not stay overnight with any other person unless accompanied by Mr or Mrs Aubrey.

Arrangements for ending placement
1 If Mr and Mrs Aubrey request the placement to end, there must be time for a planned introduction to the next placement.
2 The local authority may not remove Susan without permission of the court unless implementing child protection procedures.

Dissatisfactions and changes
These can be discussed at reviews (one and three months), or with Jayne at visits. If Mr and Mrs Aubrey feel that their concerns are not being acted upon they can implement the formal complaints procedure of which they have already been apprised.

What happens if the aims of the placement are not achieved
1 If the placement is in danger of disrupting the matter can be brought back to the court for 'directions'.
2 If the placement is not successful the local authority will seek to place the sibling group with long-term carers and until such time as they are well established they should be the youngest members of the family group.

signed by: Social worker
                    Team manager
                    Mr and Mrs Aubrey
                    Natural mother
Copies also circulated to: Local authority solicitor
                    Guardian *ad litem*
                    Solicitor of Mr and Mrs Aubrey
                    Solicitor of natural mother

Agency context

For practitioners to feel empowered and for the approach to make a difference beyond the interaction between individual worker and user, practice must be underpinned by a clear organizational value base. This involves encouraging agency debates on how commitment to empowerment, partnership and anti-oppressive practice can be expressed in policies and practice, and developing clear procedures for user involvement and for negotiating practice dilemmas such as rights versus risks. However, agencies may be part of the problem, either committed in principle but without strategies or not endorsing the principles.

The questions to debate are clear. What are the constraints and opportunities for this agency regarding empowerment, partnership and anti-oppressive practice? Who are the key people to engage and who has the power to promote such practice? What gaps in service provision exist? How might the agency promote anti-oppressive practice whilst meeting its statutory obligations – for instance, user groups, advocacy schemes, clear statements of perspective and policies? What alternative ways exist of understanding and tackling issues faced by users, especially structural inequalities?

Written agreements, and the principles of partnership and anti-oppressive practice, indicate that agencies must critically appraise their work with users and clarify their commitment to challenging oppression, discriminatory policies and inequalities. Such an initiative must be undertaken collectively by managers and workers with service users and their communities if barriers to change (professional power, professional vulnerability, bureaucracy, mistrust, powerlessness and hopelessness, practice dilemmas) are not to obstruct the opportunities for and benefits of change (openly discussed policies and procedures, power redistribution and relationship change, partnership at all levels of agency practice).

ACKNOWLEDGEMENTS

I would like to acknowledge and thank John Corden, Unit Organizer, East Leeds Family Service Unit, for sharing his ideas on using contracts, especially the contribution from law; Suzy Braye, Lecturer, School of Social Work, University of Manchester, for working with me on developing the use of written agreements in relation to partnership; and participants on various courses.

REFERENCES

Barber, J. (1991) *Beyond Casework*, London: Macmillan.
Barclay Committee (1982) *Social Workers, Their Role and Tasks*, London: London Institute for Social Work/Bedford Square Press.

BCCCS (1991) *Sukina – An Evaluation Report into the Circumstances Leading to her Death*, London: Bridge Child Care Consultancy Service.

Braye, S. and Preston-Shoot, M. (1992a) *Practising Social Work Law*, London: Macmillan.

Braye, S. and Preston-Shoot, M. (1992b) 'Honourable intentions: written agreements in welfare legislation', *Journal of Social Welfare and Family Law*, November 6: 511–28.

Butler-Sloss Committee (1988) *Report of the Inquiry into Child Abuse in Cleveland*, London: HMSO.

CCETSW (1991) *The Teaching of Child Care in the Diploma in Social Work*, London: Central Council for Education and Training in Social Work.

Corden, J. (1980) 'Contracts in social work practice', *British Journal of Social Work* 10(2): 143–62.

Corden, J. and Preston-Shoot, M. (1987a) *Contracts in Social Work*, Aldershot: Gower.

Corden, J. and Preston-Shoot, M. (1987b) 'Contract or con trick? A reply to Rojek and Collins', *British Journal of Social Work* 17(5): 535–43.

Corden, J. and Preston-Shoot, M. (1988) 'Contract or con trick? A postscript', *British Journal of Social Work* 18(6): 623–34.

Croft, S. and Beresford, P. (1989) 'User involvement, citizenship and social policy', *Critical Social Policy* 26, 9(2): 5–18.

DHSS (1974) *Report of the Committee of Inquiry into the Care and Supervision Provided in Relation to Maria Colwell*, London: HMSO.

DoH (1989) *The Care of Children. Principles and Practice in Regulations and Guidance*, London: HMSO.

DoH (1991a) *The Children Act 1989. Guidance and Regulations. Volume 2. Family Support, Day Care and Educational Provision for Young Children*, London: HMSO.

DoH (1991b) *Care Management and Assessment. Summary of Practice Guidance*, London: HMSO.

DoH (1991c) *The Children Act 1989. Guidance and Regulations. Volume 3. Family Placements*, London: HMSO.

DoH (1991d) *Care Management and Assessment. Practitioners' Guide*, London: HMSO.

Dominelli, L. (1988) *Anti-Racist Social Work*, London: Macmillan.

Francis, M. (1988) 'The skeleton in the cupboard: experiential geneogram work for family therapy trainees', *Journal of Family Therapy* 10(2):135–52.

Goodman Report (1990) *Report of the Inquiry into the Death of a Child in Care*, Derbyshire and Nottinghamshire County Councils and Area Child Protection Committees.

Hanmer, J. and Statham, D. (1988) *Women and Social Work: Towards a Woman Centred Practice*, London: Macmillan.

Illich, I. (1975) *Medical Nemesis – The Expropriation of Health*, London: Calder and Boyars.

Lee, J. (1991) 'Empowerment through mutual aid groups: a practice grounded conceptual framework', *Groupwork* 4(1): 5–21.

Levy, A. and Kahan, B. (1991) *The Pin Down Experience and the Protection of Children. The Report of the Staffordshire Child Care Inquiry, 1990*, Staffordshire County Council.

Maluccio, A. and Simm, M. (1989) 'The use of agreements in foster family placements', in J. Aldgate, A. Maluccio and C. Reeves (eds) *Adolescents in Foster Families*, London: Batsford.

Mistry, T. and Brown, A. (1991) 'Black/white co-working in groups', *Groupwork* 4(2): 101–18.

Mullender, A. (1991) 'Nottingham advocacy group: giving a voice to the users of mental health services', *Practice* 5(1): 5–12.

Mullender, A. and Ward, D. (1991) *Self-Directed Groupwork: Users Take Action for Empowerment*, London: Whiting and Birch.

Nelken, D. (1987) 'The use of 'contracts' as a social work technique', *Current Legal Problems* 40: 207–32.

Phillimore, P. (1982) 'Some comments on the interpretation of clienthood', *FSU Quarterly* 26: 37–43.

Phillipson, J. (1992) *Practising Equality. Women, Men and Social Work*, London: CCETSW.

Preston-Shoot, M. and Agass, D. (1990) *Making Sense of Social Work: Psychodynamics, Systems and Practice*, London: Macmillan.

Pugh, G. and De'Ath, E. (1989) *Working Towards Partnership in the Early Years*, London: National Children's Bureau.

Rees, S. (1991) *Achieving Power. Practice and Policy in Social Welfare*, North Sydney: Allen and Unwin.

Rojek, C. and Collins, S. (1987) 'Contract or con trick?' *British Journal of Social Work* 17(2): 199–211.

Smale, G. (1983) 'Can we afford not to develop social work practice?' *British Journal of Social Work* 13(3): 251–64.

Social Services Inspectorate (1991) *Getting the Message Across: A Guide to Developing and Communicating Policies, Principles and Procedures on Assessment*, London: HMSO.

Stratton, P., Preston-Shoot, M. and Hanks, H. (1990) *Family Therapy: Training and Practice*, Birmingham: Venture Press.

Wilcox, R., Smith, D., Moore, J., Hewitt, A., Allan, G., Walker, H., Ropata, M., Monu, L. and Featherstone, T. (1991) *Family Decision Making. Family Group Conferences: Practitioners' Views*, New Zealand: Practitioners' Publishing.

FURTHER READING

Aldgate, J. (ed.) (1989) *Using Written Agreements with Children and Families*, London: Family Rights Group.

FRG (1991) *The Children Act 1989 – An FRG Briefing Pack*, London: Family Rights Group.

Macdonald, S. (1991) *All Equal Under The Act?*, London: Race Equality Unit/National Institute for Social Work.

Preston-Shoot, M. (1989a) 'Using contracts in groupwork', *Groupwork* 2(1): 36–47.

Preston-Shoot, M. (1989b) 'A contractual approach to practice teaching', *Social Work Education* 8(3): 3–15.

Smith, G. and Corden, J. (1981) 'The introduction of contracts in a Family Service Unit', *British Journal of Social Work* 11(3): 289–314.

Name index

Subject index

Printed and bound by CPI Group (UK) Ltd, Croydon, CR0 4YY

01/11/2024

01782616-0001